Medicines Use Reviews

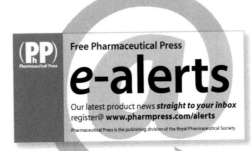

Medicines Use Reviews
A practical guide

Susan Youssef MRPharmS, PgDip (clinical pharmacy)
Senior Lecturer in Pharmacy Practice,
De Montfort University Leicester, UK
Community Pharmacist Manager, UK

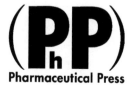

Pharmaceutical Press

Published by the Pharmaceutical Press
1 Lambeth High Street, London SE1 7JN, UK

(**P.P**) is a trade mark of Pharmaceutical Press

Pharmaceutical Press is the publishing division of the Royal
Pharmaceutical Society of Great Britain

First published 2010

Typeset by Thomson Digital, Noida, India
Printed in Great Britain by TJ International, Padstow, Cornwall
Index provided by Indexing Specialists, Hove, East Sussex, UK

ISBN 978 0 85369 887 6

Contents

Preface

The advent of the new Community Pharmacy Contract in April 2005 introduced the advanced service, Medicine Use Review (MUR) service and the Prescription Intervention service. The MUR service requires pharmacist and pharmacy accreditation. Following accreditation, the pharmacist can invite suitable patients for MURs to assess their compliance and concordance with their prescribed medication regimen.

MURs have allowed pharmacists to develop closer relationships with their patients and to have a greater understanding of their medical conditions. Building closer relationships with patients leads to patients placing greater trust in their community pharmacists. Along with this comes an array of questions and concerns from patients about their prescribed medicines, with the community pharmacist increasingly becoming the source of the answers.

This book provides pharmacists with a guide on how to conduct successful MURs for specific medical conditions. This book consists of 10 chapters, each containing subchapters on specific medical conditions and is intended for use as a quick reference guide. The aim is to provide an evidence-based approach to the treatment options available for each medical condition, along with additional considerations for discussion with patients during MURs. An ideal time to glance at the book is immediately before inviting a patient for an MUR. Assembly of their prescription can guide pharmacists as to which chapter they will need to read.

Although MURs focus on medicines, there is scope for the community pharmacist to exercise a role in promoting healthy lifestyles and a signpost to other services that benefit patients. It is hoped that *Medicines Use Reviews: A practical guide* will raise the standard of practice in community pharmacy and allow the provision of higher-quality advice during MURs. If this is achieved then the profile of the profession will ultimately be raised.

Susan Youssef

January 2010

Acknowledgements

I wish to express my thanks to Sandra Hall, Head of Pharmacy Practice at the Leicester School of Pharmacy, for reading the manuscript and offering helpful comments.

My most sincere thanks go to my family, particularly my husband, Haney, for his continual support and encouragement. Finally I thank my 3-year-old son Daniel for being a constant source of pleasure and entertainment while writing this book.

About the author

Susan Youssef registered as a pharmacist in 2002, having completed her degree at Leicester School of Pharmacy. Susan completed a split pre-registration training year in hospital and community sectors and progressed to become a pharmacist manager for Dean and Smedley Pharmacy in 2003. She completed her Postgraduate Diploma in Clinical Pharmacy (Community) in 2005 and Postgraduate Certificate of Community Pharmacy Management in 2006. Susan achieved her Practice Certificate in Medicine Use Reviews in 2005 and has developed her role in community pharmacy with a research interest in Medicine Use Reviews. In 2007 Susan was appointed as a senior lecturer in pharmacy practice at the Leicester School of Pharmacy.

Introduction

The advanced service of Medicine Use Review (MUR) is aimed at helping patients to use their medicines more effectively. The service aims to improve patients' concordance, knowledge and use of their medicines by:

- establishing patients' understanding and actual use of their medicines
- identifying, discussing and resolving poor or ineffective use of their medicines
- identifying adverse effects and drug interactions that may affect patient compliance
- improving the clinical and cost-effectiveness of prescribed medicines and reducing medicine wastage.[1,2]

Service specification and pharmacy premises accreditation

MURs are normally carried out face to face with the patient in the community pharmacy. The pharmacy where MURs are conducted must have a designated consultation area, which should also allow confidential consultations to be carried out. Both the patient and the pharmacist should be able to sit down together and speak at normal volumes without being overheard.[1,2] The consultation area may also benefit from having a table and space for a computer. Once the consultation area is installed the pharmacy needs to self-certify that it meets the requirements. This can be done using the PSNC's PREM1 Premises Self-certification form which is submitted to the local primary care trust (PCT).[1]

MURs can be carried out in other locations, e.g. in the patient's home, but approval from the primary care organisation must be sought before providing this service. In this case the pharmacist is required to complete the PSNC's PREM2 Application for consent to conduct MUR away from pharmacy form and submit it to the local PCT.[1]

Pharmacist accreditation

Registered pharmacists providing a MUR service will need to be accredited to do so. The accreditation process involves successful completion of a course and assessment offered by a higher education institution. The assessment framework consists of three main elements: clinical and pharmaceutical knowledge; accessing and applying information; and documentation and referral. The three assessment framework elements incorporate five main competencies. Each of the five competencies is linked to a series of behavioural indicators that form the basis of the assessment. The five competencies are to:

1. demonstrate relevant clinical and pharmaceutical knowledge to deliver MURs, taking into account patients' individual needs
2. demonstrate the ability to identify and make recommendations around therapeutic issues relating to patient safety, clinical benefit and cost-effectiveness
3. demonstrate the ability to identify, access, evaluate and use available written sources of information
4. demonstrate the ability to reach a shared agreement with patients
5. ensure that recommendations agreed with the patient are documented and appropriately communicated in a timely manner.[2]

Once accreditation has been obtained, a copy of the certificate must be provided to the primary care organisation before commencing the MUR service provision.[1]

Who do you invite for an MUR?

MURs can be conducted on patients every 12 months. The MUR can be conducted only on patients who have been using the pharmacy for the dispensing of their prescriptions for the previous 3 months. The patient must be taking multiple medications. Suitable patient groups include patients with long-term conditions or those on multiple medicines. Primary care organisations may identify particular patient groups who would be appropriate for targeting.[2]

A pharmacy is currently permitted to provide 400 MURs during the year 1 April to 31 March.[1]

The MUR form

The MUR and any recommendations should be sent to the patient's general practitioner (GP) using the nationally agreed template only in cases where action could be necessary by them. If there are no action points following the MUR, the pharmacist is required to inform the GP that the patient attended the MUR at the pharmacy.

A copy of the MUR summary and recommendations should also be given to the patient. A record of the MUR should also be made on the patient's pharmacy record (Figure 1).[1,2]

It is advisable to keep the MUR form for a period of 2 years or as long as the primary care organisation requires.[1] Further consideration of storage of paper MUR forms at the pharmacy must be borne in mind. It may be worthwhile investing in a filing cabinet or bookcase! Some pharmacy software systems are capable of producing and storing electronic MUR forms. Storage of MUR forms becomes less of an issue in this case.

MUR form documentation

Interventions that may be made and recorded on the MUR form include the following:

- Advice on medicines use
- Checking patients' technique and use of medicine dosage forms, e.g. inhaler devices
- Advice given on adverse effects from medication
- Advice given on any practical problems in ordering, obtaining, taking and using medicines
- Identifying any medicines that the patient is no longer taking

NHS Community Pharmacy Medicines Use Review & Prescription Intervention Service

Sheet ___ of ___   CONFIDENTIAL

Patient:
☐ For information only – no action required
☐ Follow your actions agreed below
☐ Please note the recommendations made to your GP
This is your copy of the form. You may wish to show it to other health care professionals.

GP:
☐ For information only – no action required
☐ Please consider the recommendations proposed below
A copy of the consultation record sheet can be obtained from the pharmacy if required.
Clinical codes: Medicines Use Review done by community pharmacist:
4byte:8BMF Version 2: 8BMF . Clinical Terms Version 3(Read): SNOMED-CT:1983910000000102

Patient details

Title:	First Name:		Surname:	
NHS Number:		Tel:		Date of Birth:
Address:				

Name of other people present

Consent for MUR obtained:
Oral ☐ Written ☐

GP details

GP Name:
Practice Name:
Address:
Date of review:

Review type:
Annual MUR ☐ Intervention MUR ☐

Review identified or requested by:
Pharmacist ☐ Patient ☐ Other: ☐

Location of review if not in pharmacy:

PCO permission granted for off-site MUR:
Yes ☐

Action plan

Issue	Recommendation	For consideration by:
		☐ Patient ☐ Pharmacist ☐ GP ☐ Other:
		☐ Patient ☐ Pharmacist ☐ GP ☐ Other:
		☐ Patient ☐ Pharmacist ☐ GP ☐ Other:
		☐ Patient ☐ Pharmacist ☐ GP ☐ Other:
		☐ Patient ☐ Pharmacist ☐ GP ☐ Other:

Pharmacy details

Pharmacist Name:		Pharmacist registration no.:		Pharmacy Name:			
Address:					Tel:		Email address:

Overview page   This review is based on information available to the Pharmacist held on the pharmacy Patient Medication Record system and from information provided by the patient

Figure 1 The MUR form.[1]

NHS Community Pharmacy Medicines Use Review & Prescription Intervention Service

| | | Sheet of | CONFIDENTIAL |

| Title: | First name: | Surname: | NHS Number: | Date of birth: | Date of review: |

Current Medicines (including over the counter & complementary therapies)	Does the patient use the medicine as prescribed?	Does the patient know why they are using the medicine?	More info provided on use of medicine	Is the formulation appropriate?	Are side effects reported by the patient?	General comments relating to advice, side effects and other issues
1 Name/Dosage form/Strength: Dose:	☐ Yes If no, specify:	Yes ☐ No ☐	Yes ☐ No ☐	Yes ☐ No ☐	Yes ☐ No ☐	
2 Name/Dosage form/Strength: Dose:	☐ Yes If no, specify:	Yes ☐ No ☐	Yes ☐ No ☐	Yes ☐ No ☐	Yes ☐ No ☐	
3 Name/Dosage form/Strength: Dose:	☐ Yes If no, specify:	Yes ☐ No ☐	Yes ☐ No ☐	Yes ☐ No ☐	Yes ☐ No ☐	
4 Name/Dosage form/Strength: Dose:	☐ Yes If no, specify:	Yes ☐ No ☐	Yes ☐ No ☐	Yes ☐ No ☐	Yes ☐ No ☐	
5 Name/Dosage form/Strength: Dose:	☐ Yes If no, specify:	Yes ☐ No ☐	Yes ☐ No ☐	Yes ☐ No ☐	Yes ☐ No ☐	
6 Name/Dosage form/Strength: Dose:	☐ Yes If no, specify:	Yes ☐ No ☐	Yes ☐ No ☐	Yes ☐ No ☐	Yes ☐ No ☐	

Consultation record This review is based on information available to the Pharmacist held on the pharmacy Patient Medication Record system and from information provided by the patient

Figure 1 *(continued)*

- Identifying any need for a change of dosage form to facilitate effective medicine usage
- Recommendations for changing generic medicines to branded products when clinically appropriate and vice versa
- Proposals for dose optimisation, e.g. in cases where a patient has been prescribed multiple doses of a lower-strength product when a higher-strength version is available
- Suggestions to improve clinical effectiveness.[1,2]

Additional suggestions for documentation on the MUR form include:

- Any aspect of public health, e.g. the patient's smoking status, weight or exercise regimen
- If the patient is compliant with the prescribed regimen, document this in the action plan section of the form
- Document any signposting information provided to the patient during the MUR, e.g. information provided on specialist support groups
- Over-the-counter (OTC) medication that is used regularly.

If recommendations are made during the MUR, ensure that diplomacy is used on the MUR form so as not to appear as a strict instruction to the GP. Thus the use of phrases such as 'please consider' or 'if felt appropriate' may not leave the GP wanting to put the MUR form in the shredder!

It is also important to remember that patients will receive a copy of the MUR so avoid using terminology or abbreviations that they will not understand, e.g. the use of 'od' instead of writing 'once daily'.[1]

Communication skills

MURs are a patient-focused service requiring good communication skills. The core elements to good communication skills are:

- listening with the intent to understand
- checking patients' understanding using open and closed questioning to elicit information
- maintaining good eye contact

- creating rapport
- speaking clearly
- using body language appropriately.[3]

Possible barriers to patients receiving information during an MUR may include:

- not listening
- misunderstanding
- ignoring information
- making judgements about information provided
- the environment in the consultation area, e.g. the position of seating
- interruptions
- understanding ethnic, cultural and religious issues
- inappropriate use of body language or tone of voice by the speaker.[3]

There are also possible barriers to pharmacists delivering effective communication. Some of these include:

- giving too much or not enough information
- giving the wrong information or conflicting advice
- not speaking clearly
- using language that the patient cannot understand.[3]

It is also important to remember that certain patient groups, e.g. elderly people, may be hard of hearing and may feel that it is impolite to ask questions.

Overcoming barriers to MURs

It is well recognised that there are barriers to MUR service provision. Suggestions for overcoming existing barriers to MUR service provision are discussed below.

Working in a busy dispensary

The staff skill mix will determine whether certain dispensing processes and responsibilities can be delegated. Improving the skill mix ensures that the pharmacy operates smoothly while the pharmacist is in the consultation room. Time management can be improved by recording the dispensary's activities on an hourly basis in order to monitor which of these can be delegated.[4] Effectively communicating with the public on prescription waiting times and increasing the prescription collection service are ways to improve control over the dispensary workload.

Opportunistic MUR versus an appointment system

- Opportunistic MURs may be more advantageous than an appointment system, as the patient is already in the pharmacy waiting for the prescription to be dispensed. In this instance it is reasonable to ask the dispensing technician to prepare the prescription while the pharmacist conducts the MUR.
- An appointment system is beneficial if the option of conducting MURs is feasible during consistently quiet periods of time in the pharmacy.[4] An appointment system may also allow the pharmacist to invite patients who may require a longer period of time for their MURs or complex patients who may be taking a large number of medicines. It is advisable to have appointment cards to give to the patients and to remind them of their appointments. It is worth bearing in mind that, despite a conscious effort to conduct an appointment system at the pharmacy, there will be a proportion of patients who will not attend. The pharmacy's telephone number on the appointment card may encourage patients to inform of their non-attendance. The pharmacy could also ring the patient the day before the appointment to confirm attendance.

Engaging pharmacy staff

Training the team ensures that they understand the process and can be involved in identifying and inviting potential patients for MURs. Practising an MUR on a member of the pharmacy staff will provide the pharmacist with valuable experience and allows the pharmacy staff member to understand the process and the benefits to the patient. As a result the pharmacy staff can promote the service at the pharmacy. After all, the medicine counter assistants are the first point of contact for patients at the pharmacy!

Engaging local GP practices

It is vital to contact local GP practices to inform them of the MUR service provision at the pharmacy. This can be in the form of a visit or letter to the practice. GP views on MURs are varied but some examples of their opinions on what constitutes a useful MUR include:

- receiving information on patients who have compliance problems or where there are issues relating to adverse effects or interactions
- the pharmacist ensuring that patients understand more about their medicines
- having a closer working relationship with the practice.[5]

Meeting with GPs can help them understand the MUR process and may also be an opportunity to encourage GPs to refer patients to the pharmacy. This may also be an ideal time to discuss how MURs may benefit the GP practice.

Perceived lack of benefit to patients

Patients may not appreciate the need for a review at the pharmacy especially as they are more used to a 6-monthly or annual review at the GP practice. Some patients may feel that the pharmacist is encroaching on the GP's role and may refuse to participate in the MUR. A reluctance to participate may also be attributed to a limited understanding of the MUR process. Good communication with the patient, which focuses on the benefits to the patient, often results in the patient accepting the invitation for an MUR. The MUR may also act to develop the relationship between the pharmacist and the patient.

Pharmacist confidence in MUR service provision

Practice, practice and even more practice will build up confidence levels in MUR service provision! A mentoring scheme with another pharmacist who is experienced in MUR service provision may provide additional support and allows sharing of experiences. Once the basics have been accomplished, it is interesting to focus on patients with specific conditions, e.g. patients who have asthma or diabetes, and develop a structured approach to your MURs. Regular continuing professional development (CPD) is an important factor in increasing confidence levels.

References

1. Pharmaceutical Services Negotiating Committee. Advanced Services. Available at: www.psnc.org.uk/pages/advanced_services. html (accessed 19 October 2009).
2. Department of Health. *Implementing the new Community Pharmacy Contractual Framework*. London: DH, 2005. Available at: www.dh.gov.uk/en/Publicationsandstatistics/Publications/ PublicationsPolicyAndGuidance/DH_4109256 (accessed 19 October 2009).
3. Communication in Healthcare. Available at: www.healthcare skills.nhs.uk/commskills.html (accessed 28 March 2009).
4. Wang LN.How to make a success of MURs. *Pharm J 2007; 278: 315–18.*
5. Wilcock M, Harding G.General practitioners' perceptions of medicines use reviews by pharmacists. *Pharm J 2007; 279: 501–3.*

1
Gastrointestinal conditions

Gastro-oesophageal reflux disease

Condition

Gastro-oesophageal reflux disease (GORD) is a condition where there is reflux of the gastroduodenal contents into the oesophagus, causing symptoms of heartburn and acid regurgitation.

Treatment options

Antacids and alginates, H_2-receptor antagonists, proton pump inhibitors (PPIs) and motility stimulants (domperidone and metoclopramide).[1,2]

> **MUR tips**
>
> **Antacids and alginates (e.g. aluminium hydroxide, magnesium trisilicate, sodium alginate)**
>
> They require frequent administration, which can lead to poor compliance. During the Medicines Use Review (MUR), check how often the patient is using the antacid. Antacids are best

taken between meals and at bedtime, as symptoms are often worse at these times.[1] Aluminium-containing antacids can cause aluminium accumulation in patients with impaired renal function, so they are best avoided. They tend to be constipating whereas magnesium-containing antacids may have a laxative effect. Antacids and alginates can have a high sodium content, so care is needed in patients who require a sodium-restricted diet (e.g. patients with heart failure). Antacids can impair the absorption of some drugs such as some ACE (angiotensin-converting enzyme) inhibitors, antibacterials, bisphosphonates, iron salts and possibly levothyroxine, so patients should be advised to avoid taking antacids at the same time as the other medicines.[1]

H_2-receptor antagonists (e.g. ranitidine, nizatidine)

Generally well tolerated, although can cause headaches and dizziness. Check that patients are on the appropriate maintenance dose (Table 1.1). Cimetidine is rarely prescribed because it has a higher risk of drug interactions (due to inhibition of cytochrome P450 enzymes in the liver).[2]

Table 1.1 Maintenance doses of H_2-receptor antagonists[1,2]

H_2-receptor antagonist	Usual maintenance dose (mg twice daily)
Ranitidine	150 or 300 mg at night
Famotidine	20–40
Nizatidine	150–300

Proton pump inhibitors (e.g. omeprazole, lansoprazole)

Generally well tolerated although can cause headaches and dizziness. Check that patients are on the appropriate maintenance dose (Table 1.2). During the MUR assess whether patients still require a full dose of PPI and whether they are still symptomatic. Patients should be encouraged to step down or stop PPI treatment in the long-term management of their condition.[3] During the MUR explore how well controlled patients' symptoms are. For patients unable to take capsules, omeprazole and lansoprazole are available as orodispersible formulations. The higher cost of these formulations should be considered before routine recommendation on the MUR form.

Table 1.2 Maintenance doses of proton pump inhibitors[1]

Proton pump inhibitor	Usual maintenance daily dose (mg)
Omeprazole	20
Lansoprazole	15–30
Pantoprazole	20
Rabeprazole	10–20
Esomeprazole	20

Motility stimulants (e.g. domperidone, metoclopramide)

Often used in patients whose symptoms are not relieved by H_2-receptor antagonists or PPIs. Long-term use should be avoided to minimise adverse effects, e.g. extrapyramidal effects associated with metoclopramide. Extrapyramidal adverse effects include acute dystonic reactions involving facial and skeletal muscle spasms.[1] Metoclopramide should not be used in young adults (under the age of 20 years)[2] because extrapyramidal adverse effects are more commonly experienced in this age group.[1]

Additional considerations

- Check other medications that the patient may be taking. Use of non-steroidal anti-inflammatory drugs (NSAIDs) can cause gastric irritation if used without a suitable gastroprotective agent.
- Offer patients advice on lifestyle measures such as healthy eating.[3]
- Advise patients to avoid substances that precipitate their symptoms, e.g. smoking, alcohol, coffee, chocolate and fatty foods.[3] These substances are known to reduce the tone of the lower oesophageal sphincter and so make symptoms worse.
- Advise patients to avoid having their main meal before going to bed.[3]
- Patients should be encouraged to maintain normal body weight (body mass index [BMI] <25).[3]
- Advise patients to stop smoking. Signpost to a smoking cessation service.[3]
- Patients can also raise the head of their bed or use extra pillows to minimise acid regurgitation.[1,3]
- If symptoms persist despite treatment and lifestyle modifications advise patients to see their GP again.

References

1. Joint Formulary Committee. *British National Formulary 57*. London: BMA and RPSGB, 2009.

2. NHS Clinical Knowledge Summaries. Clinical Topic: GORD. Available at: http://cks.library.nhs.uk/dyspepsia_proven_gord (accessed 19 October 2009).
3. National Institute for Clinical Excellence. Guidance CG 17. *Managing Dyspepsia in Adults in Primary Care: Quick reference guide.* London: NICE, 2004. Available at: www.nice.org.uk/nicemedia/pdf/CG017quickrefguide.pdf (accessed 19 October 2009).

Peptic ulcer disease

Condition

Ulceration of the stomach or duodenum is present and may be determined by endoscopic examination. The most likely cause is *Helicobacter pylori* infection or use of NSAIDs.

Treatment options

PPIs and *H. pylori* eradication therapy.[1]

MUR tips

PPIs

Examples include lansoprazole and omeprazole. Full doses of PPIs are used in peptic ulcer disease (Table 1.3) for up to 2 months.[1] Once the ulcer has healed, patients are advised to continue on maintenance doses of PPIs (see Table 1.2) as required.[1] During the MUR, assess whether the patient still requires a full dose of PPI and whether they are still symptomatic. Patients should be encouraged to step down or stop PPI treatment in long-term management of their condition.[1]

H. pylori eradication therapy

H. pylori can be detected using the ^{13}C-labelled urea breath test. Patients with a positive result require eradication therapy. Triple therapy combinations that are used for *H. pylori* eradication include:

- Clarithromycin + amoxicillin + PPI (e.g. omeprazole, lansoprazole)
- Clarithromycin + metronidazole + PPI (e.g. omeprazole, lansoprazole)
- Amoxicillin + metronidazole + PPI (e.g. omeprazole, lansoprazole).[1]

Antibiotics can interact with several medications.[2] Full doses of PPIs are used in eradication therapy (Table 1.3).[3]

Table 1.3 Full doses of proton pump inhibitors used in *Helicobacter pylori* eradication[3]

Proton pump inhibitor	Dose (mg twice daily)
Esomeprazole	20
Lansoprazole	30
Omeprazole	20
Pantoprazole	40
Rabeprazole	20

Additional considerations

- Patients taking NSAIDs who develop dyspepsia may need to stop the NSAID.[1,3] In this instance a patient should be referred to his or her GP with appropriate documentation on the MUR form.
- Patients should be encouraged to self-treat with antacids or alginates once the ulcer has healed if they are no longer symptomatic.[1] Antacids and alginates may be purchased from the pharmacy and the patient offered appropriate advice on their use.
- Advise patients to stop smoking. Signpost to a smoking cessation service.[1]
- Offer patients advice on lifestyle measures such as healthy eating.[1]
- Advise patients to avoid substances that precipitate their symptoms, e.g. smoking, alcohol, coffee, chocolate and fatty foods.[1]
- Patients should be encouraged to maintain normal body weight (BMI <25).[1]
- Patients can also raise the head of their bed or use extra pillows to minimise acid regurgitation.[1]

References

1. National Institute for Clinical Excellence. *Dyspepsia: Managing dyspepsia in adults in primary care: Quick reference guide.* NICE Guidance CG 17. London: NICE, 2004. Available at: www.nice.org.uk/nicemedia/pdf/CG017quickrefguide.pdf (accessed 19 October 2009).
2. NHS Clinical Knowledge Summaries. Clinical Topic: GORD. Available at: http://cks.library.nhs.uk/dyspepsia_proven_gord (accessed 19 October 2009).
3. Joint Formulary Committee. *British National Formulary 57.* London: BMA and RPSGB, 2009.

Inflammatory bowel disease: ulcerative colitis and Crohn's disease

Condition

Crohn's disease (CD) is a condition of inflammation of one or more patches of the gastrointestinal tract and symptoms depend on the part of the gastrointestinal tract that is affected. Ulcerative colitis (UC) is a condition where inflammation develops in the colon or rectum.

Treatment options

Aminosalicylates, corticosteroids, immunomodulators and infliximab.[1,2]

MUR tips

Aminosalicylates

A variety of aminosalicylates is available (Table 1.4). Aminosalicylates are effective in preventing relapses in patients with ulcerative colitis but not Crohn's disease.[2] Explore any possible adverse effects that the patient may be experiencing. Enema and suppository formulations are often more suitable in acute exacerbations,[3] particularly if there is inflammation of the rectum or distal colon.

Table 1.4 Aminosalicylates available and their characteristics[3]

Amino-salicylate	Site of drug release	Adverse effects	Formulations available
Mesalazine (Asacol)	Terminal ileum and in the large bowel	Nausea, diarrhoea, rashes and headache	Modified-release tablets, foam enemas and suppositories
Mesalazine (Pentasa)	Continually released from the duodenum to the rectum	Nausea, diarrhoea, rashes and headache	Modified-release tablets, enemas, sachets and suppositories
Balsalazide	A combination of mesalazine + carrier molecule which is split in the colon	Nausea, diarrhoea, rashes and headache	Capsule
Olsalazine	A combination of 5-aminosalicylate + mesalazine which is split in the colon	Nausea, diarrhoea, rashes and headache	Tablet and capsule
Sulfasalazine	A combination of sulfapyridine + mesalazine which is split in the colon	Photosen-sitisation and blood disorders	Tablets, suppositories and suspension

Corticosteroids

Chronic use of corticosteroids is not beneficial to the patient.[2] They are not often prescribed for long-term use. In cases where they may be prescribed long term the pharmacist must be aware of corticosteroid interactions with other medicines such as cardiac glycosides, diuretics and phenytoin.[1]

Immunomodulators

Examples include azathioprine which can be used in patients who are corticosteroid dependent or resistant.[2] Patients on immunomodulators are more susceptible to infections[3] due to the immunosuppression that may occur.

Infliximab

Recommended for use in patients who have not responded to azathioprine and corticosteroids and where surgery is inappropriate.[4] Patients who are receiving this treatment in hospital are given an alert card[3] to carry at all times. Patients may also develop delayed hypersensitivity reactions after treatment.[3] In this instance the patient should be referred back to his or her GP/specialist.

Additional considerations

- Aminosalicylates and their formulations are not interchangeable and should be prescribed by brand. Ensure that the patient's prescription is by brand or proprietary name.
- Patients taking sulfasalazine should be encouraged to report any bruising, bleeding or sore throats.
- Smoking cessation helps to prevent relapses in CD.[2] Signpost the patient to a smoking cessation service.

- CD patients are advised to eat a balanced diet and avoid food that upsets them. High-fibre foods such as brown bread, fruit and vegetables can cause abdominal pain so patients should be advised to avoid these foods. Probiotics are of interest in CD and aim to improve the gut microorganism environment.[2] However, there is not sufficient evidence to recommend their routine use.

References

1. Joint Formulary Committee. *British National Formulary 57*. London: BMA and RPSGB, 2009.
2. General Practice (GP) Notebook. Inflammatory bowel disease. Available at: www.gpnotebook.co.uk (accessed 19 October 2009).
3. Electronic Medicines Compendium. Asacol, Pentasa, Colazide, Dipentum, Salazopyrin, Imuran and Remicade. Available at: http://emc.medicines.org.uk/ (accessed 19 October 2009).
4. National Institute for Clinical Excellence. *Crohn's Disease – Infiximab: Summary*. NICE Guideline TA40. London: NICE, 2002. Available at: www.nice.org.uk/nicemedia/pdf/CrohnsWelshEnglishA4summary.pdf (accessed 19 October 2009).

2
Cardiovascular conditions
Angina

Condition

Angina is chest pain that occurs secondary to the inadequate delivery of oxygen to the heart muscle. This is classically felt as a crushing pain over the sternum and may radiate to the left arm.

Treatment options

Nitrates, β blockers, calcium channel blockers, potassium channel activators, antiplatelet drugs, statins and ACE (angiotensin-converting enzyme) inhibitors.[1,2] Antiplatelet drugs, statins and ACE inhibitors are used to prevent new vascular events.[1]

MUR tips

Nitrates (e.g. isosorbide mononitrate)

Check the dosing interval with the patient during the MUR. Ensure that the patient has an asymmetrical twice-daily dosing interval of nitrates to ensure a nitrate-free period (as nitrate tolerance with reduced therapeutic effects may develop), e.g. 8am and 2pm dosing is a commonly used regimen.[2,3]

β Blockers (e.g. atenolol, bisoprolol)

Check that the patient is not experiencing fatigue, coldness of the extremities, sleep disturbances, sexual disturbances (all less likely with atenolol) or a small deterioration of glucose tolerance if patient is also diabetic. A blood glucose test can be offered to patients who suspect a deterioration in their diabetes. Ensure compliance with β-blocker treatment as sudden stopping can cause exacerbation of angina.[2] A liquid preparation of atenolol is available for patients who experience difficulties in swallowing tablet formulations.

Calcium channel blockers (e.g. diltiazem, verapamil)

Patients commonly experience swollen ankles, headache, postural hypotension and facial flushing. Grapefruit juice can inhibit the metabolism of verapamil so patients should be advised to avoid drinking it. Modified-release preparations of diltiazem are not interchangeable due to bioavailability variations, so prescriptions should specify the brand to be dispensed.[2] If the prescription is not by brand then a recommendation for this can be made on the MUR form.

Potassium channel activators (e.g. nicorandil)

Patients commonly experience headache as a side effect on initiation of treatment, which may result in discontinuation of therapy. Careful dose titration may alleviate this symptom. Check that the patient is using the tablets in the blister strip within 30 days of opening as per manufacturer's instructions for use.[4]

Antiplatelet drugs (e.g. aspirin)

Check that patients are taking aspirin after food and explore any side effects of dyspepsia that they may be experiencing.

Statins (e.g. simvastatin)

Check that the patient is taking the statin at night. Cholesterol synthesis is greatest at night and the rationale for taking statins at night should be explained to the patient. Refer any patient to the GP if he or she complains of muscle pain or tenderness.

ACE Inhibitors (e.g. ramipril)

Patients can experience a persistent, troublesome, dry cough that interferes with sleep while taking medicines from this group.[2] If this is troublesome then refer the patient to the GP to consider an alternative treatment.

Additional considerations

- Patients should be encouraged to stop smoking.[2,3] Signpost smokers to the nearest smoking cessation service.
- Offer patients advice on lifestyle measures such as healthy eating.[2,3]
- Advise patients to increase the level of aerobic exercise undertaken.[3]
- Encourage patients to lose weight in order to achieve a BMI (body mass index) of <25.[3]
- Alcohol consumption should be <3 units/day for men and <2 units/day for women.[3]

References

1. Scottish Intercollegiate Guidelines Network. *Management of Stable Angina*. SIGN Guideline 96. Edinburgh: SIGN, 2007. Available at: www.sign.ac.uk/pdf/qrgchd.pdf (accessed 19 October 2009).
2. Joint Formulary Committee. *British National Formulary 57*. London: BMA and RPSGB, 2009.

3. NHS Clinical Knowledge Summaries. Clinical Topic: Angina. Available at: http://cks.library.nhs.uk/angina (accessed 19 October 2009).
4. Electronic Medicines Compendium. Ikorel. Available at: http://emc.medicines.org.uk/ (accessed 19 October 2009).

Heart failure

Condition

Heart failure is a complex syndrome in which the ability of the heart to function as a pump to support a physiological circulation is impaired.

Treatment options

ACE inhibitors, loop diuretics, aldosterone antagonists, cardiac glycosides, angiotensin II antagonists and β blockers.[1–3]

MUR tips

ACE inhibitors (e.g. ramipril, lisinopril)

Cough is common in patients with heart failure due to possible coexisting smoking-related lung disease,[3] heart failure and the adverse effects of ACE inhibitors. If a patient experiences a persistent, troublesome, dry cough that interferes with sleep while taking an ACE inhibitor then refer to the GP for consideration of an alternative drug. This should be documented on the MUR form.

Loop diuretics (e.g. furosemide)

Large doses can be ototoxic so check that patients do not experience deterioration in their hearing. Patients may complain of the potent diuretic effect, which can stop them from carrying out their daily activities. Patients may also feel light-headed or dizzy while on diuretic therapy.[3] If this is the case, a blood pressure check is appropriate, and can be done during the MUR. The blood pressure result should be recorded on the MUR form.

Aldosterone antagonists

Spironolactone may increase serum potassium levels (this is less likely with lower doses). Other possible adverse effects associated with use may include electrolyte disturbances, leg cramps and gynaecomastia, which is dose related.[4] Patients should have serum urea, electrolytes and creatinine checked every 6 months if the condition is stable.[1] Check that the patient regularly attends appointments for blood tests.

Cardiac glycosides

Digoxin has a narrow therapeutic window. Some drugs can increase digoxin levels when administered concomitantly, e.g. amiodarone, erythromycin, omeprazole and tetracyclines. If a patient experiences nausea, vomiting, tachycardia, diarrhoea or confusion then suspect digoxin toxicity and refer the patient to the GP.

Angiotensin II antagonists (e.g. candesartan, valsartan)

Renal function should be monitored regularly.[3] Check that the patient is having regular blood tests and blood pressure monitoring.

β Blockers (e.g. bisoprolol and carvedilol)

Check that the patient is not experiencing fatigue, coldness of the extremities, sleep disturbances, sexual disturbances or a small deterioration of glucose tolerance if the patient is also diabetic. A blood glucose test can be offered to patients who suspect deterioration in their diabetes. Regular blood pressure monitoring is required with β blockers.[3] This can be offered during the MUR.

Additional considerations

- Alcohol consumption should be ≤3 units/day for men and ≤2 units/day for women.[2]
- Patients should be encouraged to stop smoking. Signpost smokers to a smoking cessation service.[2]
- Patients should regularly undertake low-intensity physical activity.[2]
- Patients should be advised to limit their daily salt intake to <6 g/day and not to use 'low-salt' substitutes due to their high potassium content.[2]
- Patients should be encouraged to weigh themselves regularly at a set time each day. Any weight gain of more than 1.5–2 kg over 2 days should be reported to their GP as it may be an indicator of worsening heart failure.[2]

References

1. National Institute for Clinical Excellence. *Chronic Heart Failure: Management of chronic heart failure in adults in primary and secondary care.* NICE Guideline CG 5. London: NICE, 2003. Available at: www.nice.org.uk/nicemedia/pdf/CG5NICEguideline.pdf (accessed 19 October 2009).
2. Scottish Intercollegiate Guidelines Network. *Management of Chronic Heart Failure.* SIGN Guideline 95. Edinburgh: SIGN, 2007. Available at: www.sign.ac.uk/pdf/qrgchd.pdf (accessed 19 October 2009).

3. NHS Clinical Knowledge Summaries. Clinical Topic: Heart Failure. Available at: http://cks.library.nhs.uk/heart_failure (accessed 19 October 2009).
4. Electronic Medicines Compendium. Aldactone. Available at: http://emc.medicines.org.uk (accessed 19 October 2009).

Hypertension

Condition

Hypertension is a sustained systolic blood pressure ≥140 mmHg and sustained diastolic blood pressure ≥90 mmHg.

Treatment options

Thiazide diuretics, calcium channel blockers, ACE inhibitors, angiotensin II antagonists and α blockers.[1]

MUR tips

Thiazides (e.g. bendroflumethiazide)

First-line treatment for patients aged over 55 years and black patients of any age.[2] Adverse effects associated with use include electrolyte disturbances (especially hypokalaemia), altered lipid concentration, exacerbation of diabetes, hyperuricaemia and gout.[3] Any patient reporting adverse effects should be encouraged to contact his or her GP. The referral can also be documented on the MUR form.

Calcium channel blockers (e.g. amlodipine, felodipine)

First-line treatment for patients aged over 55 years and black patients of any age.[2] Patients commonly experience swollen ankles, headache, postural hypotension and facial flushing. Grapefruit juice can inhibit the metabolism of some calcium channel blockers (e.g. felodipine, lacidipine)[3] so patients are advised to avoid drinking it.

ACE inhibitors (e.g. lisinopril, ramipril)

First-line treatment in patients aged under 55 years.[2] If a patient experiences a persistent, troublesome, dry cough that interferes with sleep while taking medicines from this group then refer to his or her GP.[1]

Angiotensin II antagonists (e.g. losartan, valsartan)

These are considered for first-line use in patients aged under 55 years who are intolerant of ACE inhibitors.[2] Adverse effects associated with use are usually mild and may include hypotension and dizziness.[3] Check that the patient has regular blood pressure monitoring.

α Blockers (e.g. doxazosin, prazosin)

First-dose postural hypotension may occur, particularly in elderly people.[1] Patients are advised to take the dose at bedtime. Other adverse effects associated with use may include dizziness, fatigue and oedema.[3]

Additional considerations

- Advise patients to reduce their salt intake to <6 g/day.[2,4]
- Antacids and alginates can have a high sodium content so encourage awareness of this during the MUR.[3]

- Alcohol consumption should be ≤3 units/day for men and ≤2 units/day for women.[4]
- Patients should be encouraged to stop smoking. Signpost smokers to a smoking cessation service.[2]
- A pharmacy blood pressure-monitoring service can be offered to the patient.
- Encourage patients to take regular aerobic physical exercise for ≥30 min/day, ideally on most days but on at least 3 days of the week.[4]
- Patients should be encouraged to maintain normal body weight (BMI <25).[4]
- Patients should consume at least five portions per day of fresh fruit and vegetables[4] (Table 2.1).
- Advise patients to reduce the intake of total and saturated fat in their diet.[4]

Table 2.1 Examples of one portion size of fruit and vegetables[5]

Fruit and vegetables	Examples of one portion size
Fresh fruit	2 plums, 1 apple, 1 orange, 7 strawberries, 14 cherries, 2 kiwi fruit, half a grapefruit, 1 pear, 3 apricots
Dried fruits	1 tablespoon of raisins, currants, sultanas, 2 figs, 3 prunes
Fruit juices	150mL of 100% juice, e.g. fruit or vegetable smoothie
Green vegetables	2 broccoli spears, 8 cauliflower florets, 4 heaped tablespoons of green beans
Salad vegetables	3 celery sticks, 4 cm piece of cucumber, 1 medium tomato

Table 2.1 *Continued*

Fruit and vegetables	Examples of one portion size
Cooked, tinned and frozen vegetables	3 heaped tablespoons of carrots, peas or sweetcorn
Pulses and beans	3 heaped tablespoons of baked beans, kidney beans, haricot beans, chickpeas

References

1. NHS Clinical Knowledge Summaries. Clinical Topic: Hypertension. Available at: http://cks.library.nhs.uk/hypertension (accessed 19 October 2009).
2. National Institute for Health and Clinical Excellence. *Hypertension: Management of hypertension in adults in primary care: A quick reference guide.* NICE Guideline CG 34. London: NICE, 2006. Available at: www.nice.org.uk/nicemedia/pdf/cg034quickrefguide.pdf (accessed 19 October 2009).
3. Joint Formulary Committee. *British National Formulary 57.* London: BMA and RPSGB, 2009.
4. Williams B, Poulter NR, Brown MJ, *et al.* British Hypertension Society guidelines for hypertension management 2004 (BHS-IV): summary. *BMJ* 2004; 328: 634–40. Available at: www.bhsoc.org/pdfs/Summary%20Guidelines%202004.pdf (accessed 19 October 2009).
5. NHS. 5 a day. Available at: www.5aday.nhs.uk/WhatCounts/PortionSizes.aspx (accessed 19 October 2009).

Hyperlipidaemia

Condition

Hyperlipidaemia is elevated concentrations of any or all of the lipids in the plasma.

Treatment options

Statins, fibrates, nicotinic acid and ezetimibe.[1]

MUR tips

Statins (e.g. atorvastatin, simvastatin, pravastatin)

Check that the patient is taking the statin at night (except for atorvastatin which can be taken at any time of the day).[2] Cholesterol synthesis is greatest at night and the rationale for taking statins at night should be explained to the patient. Refer any patients to their GP if they complain of muscle pain, tenderness or weakness, especially if associated with fever or malaise.[1,3] Patients who take concomitant medications that are metabolised by the cytochrome P450 liver enzyme system are advised to take pravastatin (which is not significantly metabolised by the cytochrome P450 system) as the preferred lipid-lowering treatment.[1,2] Patients should be advised to avoid the consumption of grapefruit juice while taking statins.

Grapefruit juice can increase plasma concentrations of atorvastatin and simvastatin which may lead to unwanted adverse effects.[3]

Fibrates (e.g. bezafibrate)

Patients who have hypertriglyceridaemia are considered for treatment with fibrates.[1,3] Adverse effects associated with use may include loss of appetite, nausea and feelings of fullness in the stomach which are often transient.[2]

Nicotinic acid

Patients who have hypertriglyceridaemia are considered for treatment with nicotinic acid.[1] Adverse effects associated with use may include flushing episodes, dyspepsia, diarrhoea, nausea and abdominal pain.[2] Nicotinic acid should be used with caution in patients with a history of peptic ulceration.[3]

Ezetimibe

This is recommended as monotherapy for adults with primary heterozygous, familial or non-familial hypercholesterolaemia.[4] Adverse effects associated with use may include headache, fatigue and gastrointestinal disturbances.[2]

Additional considerations

- Encourage patients to have a diet low in saturated fats. Saturated fats should be replaced by mono-unsaturated and polyunsaturated fats.[5]
- Encourage patients to eat five portions of fruit and vegetables per day[5] (see Table 2.1).
- Encourage patients to eat two portions of fish per week; one portion should be an oily fish.[5]

- Patients are advised to do 30 min of moderate intensity exercise on at least 5 days per week.[5]
- Patients should be encouraged to maintain normal body weight (BMI <25).[5]
- Alcohol consumption should be ≤3 units/day for men and ≤2 units/day for women.[5]
- Patients should be encouraged to stop smoking. Signpost smokers to a smoking cessation service.[5]

References

1. Scottish Intercollegiate Guidelines Network. *Risk Estimation and the Prevention of Cardiovascular Disease.* SIGN Guideline 97. Edinburgh: SIGN, 2007. Available at: www.sign.ac.uk/pdf/qrgchd. pdf (accessed 19 October 2009).
2. Electronic Medicines Compendium. Lipitor, Lipostat, Ezetrol and Niaspan. Available at: http://emc.medicines.org.uk/ (accessed 19 October 2009).
3. Joint Formulary Committee. *British National Formulary 57.* London: BMA and RPSGB, 2009.
4. National Institute for Health and Clinical Excellence. *Hypercholesterolaemia – Ezetimibe: A quick reference guide.* NICE Guideline TA132. London: NICE, 2007. Available at: www.nice. org.uk/nicemedia/pdf/TA132QRGFINAL.pdf (accessed 19 October 2009).
5. National Institute for Health and Clinical Excellence. *Lipid Modification: A quick reference guide.* NICE Guideline CG 67. London: NICE, 2008. Available at: www.nice.org.uk/nicemedia/ pdf/CG67quickrefguide.pdf (accessed 19 October 2009).

Conditions requiring anticoagulant treatment

Conditions

Some examples of conditions requiring treatment with anticoagulant agents include atrial fibrillation, calf vein thrombosis, proximal deep vein thrombosis (DVT), mechanical prosthetic heart valves, antiphospholipid syndrome and pulmonary embolus.[1]

Treatment options

Anticoagulants, e.g. warfarin.[1]

MUR Tips

Warfarin

- Check that the patient knows the indication for their warfarin treatment.
- Check that patients take the warfarin at the same time each day (usually 6pm) and know what to do if they miss a dose or accidentally take an overdose. Missed doses should never be adjusted for and patients should be advised to take the next dose at the correct time and arrange an appointment at their anticoagulation clinic to have an international normalised ratio (INR) test.

- Check that the patient regularly attends anticoagulation clinic appointments.
- Advise patients to present their anticoagulant book (yellow book) (Figure 2.1) with each prescription for warfarin. This allows the pharmacist to closely monitor INR test results and to ensure that INR results are at a safe level when dispensing prescriptions for warfarin.
- Check that the patient knows their current dose in milligrams.
- Check that patients know for how long they will be taking warfarin.[2,3]

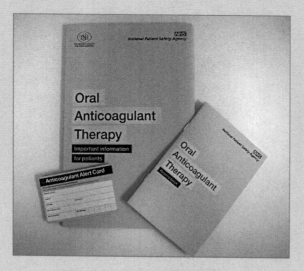

Figure 2.1   The anticoagulant book (yellow book).

Additional considerations

- Food, supplement and drug interactions with warfarin are extensive (Table 2.2). Ensure that the patient is informed of the major interactions.[3] A leaflet on food and supplement interactions can be given to the patient during the MUR.

- Advise patients of the importance of avoiding alcohol binge drinking.
- Advise patients to inform other healthcare professionals of their warfarin usage, e.g. the dentist.

Table 2.2 Some of the major interactions with warfarin[4]

Foods	Supplements	Drugs
Seaweed Cranberry juice Green leafy vegetables, e.g. spinach and broccoli if eaten in larger quantities than usual intake Papaya Soy protein products (including soya milk and tofu) Mango	Chondroitin plus glucosamine Coenzyme Q10 Devil's claw Ginkgo biloba Green tea St John's wort	Antibiotics (e.g. azithromycin, erythromycin, tetracycline) Non-steroidal anti-inflammatory drugs Stomach ulcer medicines or acid-reducing agents (e.g. cimetidine, omeprazole, ranitidine) Antidepressants (e.g. fluoxetine, paroxetine, sertraline) Lipid-lowering agents (fibrates and statins) Antifungal agents (e.g. itraconazole)

References

1. Baglin TP, Keeling DM, Watson HG, for the British Committee for Standards in Haematology. *Guidelines on Oral Anticoagulation (Warfarin)*, 3rd edn. London: British Society for Haematology, 2005: 277–86. Available at: www.bcshguidelines.com/pdf/oralan ticoagulation.pdf (accessed 19 October 2009).
2. National Patient Safety Agency. Actions that make anticoagulant therapy safer: dispensing oral anticoagulants. Patient Safety Alert 18,

2007. Available at: www.npsa.nhs.uk/nrls/alerts-and-directives/alerts/anticoagulant/ (accessed 19 October 2009).

3. Youssef S. Patients taking warfarin: Problems revealed by medicine use reviews. *Pharm J* 2008; 280: 662.

4. Health Canada. *It's your Health: Warfarin interactions with drugs, natural health and food products.* Ottawa: Health Canada. Available at: www.hc-sc.gc.ca/hl-vs/iyh-vsv/med/warfarin-eng.php (accessed 19 October 2009).

Conditions requiring antiplatelet treatment

Condition

Antiplatelet treatment is required in conditions where occlusion of blood supply may arise, e.g. stroke and myocardial infarction. Stroke can be either ischaemic (this is where a blood vessel to the brain is completely blocked) or haemorrhagic (this involves bleeding from a blood vessel in the brain). Myocardial infarction involves an occlusion of the blood supply to the heart.

Treatment options

Aspirin, clopidogrel and modified-release dipyridamole.[1]

MUR tips

Aspirin

Low-dose aspirin (75 mg daily) is recommended as long-term secondary prevention treatment.[2] During the MUR check that patients are taking aspirin with or after food and explore any possible symptoms of dyspepsia. If symptoms of dyspepsia are present it is beneficial for the patient to have an antisecretory drug (such as a proton pump inhibitor or PPI) co-prescribed until they can be switched to an alternative antiplatelet drug.[2]

In this instance a patient should be referred back to the GP for this consideration with the appropriate documentation made on the MUR form.

Clopidogrel

Is a suitable alternative for patients who do not tolerate aspirin or where aspirin is contraindicated.[2] Clopidogrel can increase bleeding time so advise patients to report excessive bleeding,[1] e.g. nose bleeds or bruising.[3] Pharmacists should also be aware that PPIs can lower the clinical effectiveness of clopidogrel.[3] Patients taking both should be referred to the GP for a review with this recommendation documented on the MUR form.

Dipyridamole modified-release capsules (Persantin Retard)

This is recommended as secondary prevention treatment following an ischaemic stroke or transient ischaemic attack (TIA).[2] Adverse effects of vomiting, diarrhoea, dizziness, hypotension, hot flushes and headache are commonly seen in the early stages of treatment.[3]

Additional considerations

Aspirin

Enteric-coated aspirin tablets have no additional benefit in gastric protection over dispersible aspirin[2] so they should not be recommended as an alternative if the patient is experiencing dyspepsia.

Dipyridamole

Patients should be reminded that once the capsule container of Persantin Retard is opened it should be discarded after 6 weeks.[3]

During the MUR check that patients are aware of this and that they do not have containers that have been open for longer than this time period.

References

1. NHS Clinical Knowledge Summaries. Clinical Topic: Stroke and TIA. Available at: http://cks.library.nhs.uk/stroke_and_tia (accessed 19 October 2009).
2. National Prescribing Centre. Prescribing antiplatelet drugs in primary care. *MeReC Bull* 2005; 15(6):21–4. Available at: www.npc.co.uk/ebt/merec/cardio/acute/resources/merec_bulletin_vol15_no6.pdf (accessed 19 October 2009).
3. Electronic Medicines Compendium. Plavix and Persantin Retard. Available at: http://emc.medicines.org.uk (accessed 19 October 2009).

Arrhythmias

Condition

Various types exist but commonly present as an irregular heartbeat which is often location dependent in the heart, e.g. atrial flutter and ventricular tachycardia.

Treatment options

Amiodarone, β blockers, disopyramide, flecainide and calcium channel blockers.[1]

MUR tips

Amiodarone

Due to its long half-life dosing is usually once daily.[1] Adverse effects associated with use include nausea and vomiting on treatment initiation, bradycardia, hypothyroidism or hyperthyroidism, corneal microdeposits, liver problems and photosensitivity.[2] During the MUR check whether the patient is attending regularly for thyroid and liver function tests during treatment.[3] Patients should also be advised to wear a high protection sunscreen product or ensure that their skin is covered to minimise photosensitivity reactions.

β Blockers

Sotalol is used for its antiarrhythmic properties. Check if the patient is experiencing any adverse effects including fatigue, coldness of the extremities, sleep disturbances, sexual disturbances or a small deterioration of glucose tolerance if patient is also diabetic. A blood glucose test can be offered to patients who suspect deterioration in their diabetes.[1]

Disopyramide

This may provoke or worsen arrhythmias especially if hypokalaemia is present. If the existing arrhythmia is exacerbated then an urgent review of disopyramide treatment is required and the patient should be referred to a GP.[2] Adverse effects that may be experienced are due to its anticholinergic effects, e.g. dry mouth, constipation and urinary retention.[2]

Flecainide

This can provoke or worsen arrhythmias in patients with structural heart disease. Adverse effects include nausea, vomiting and visual disturbances.[2]

Calcium channel blockers, e.g. verapamil

Patients commonly experience swollen ankles, headache, postural hypotension and facial flushing. Grapefruit juice can inhibit the metabolism of verapamil so patients are advised to avoid drinking it.[2]

Additional considerations

Amiodarone

- Concomitant use of stimulant laxatives (e.g. senna and bisacodyl) can cause hypokalaemia, which may lead to torsade de pointes (a rare ventricular arrhythmia that can, in turn, lead to ventricular fibrillation and sudden death in the absence of medical intervention). If a patient requests an over-the-counter preparation he or she is best advised to use other types of laxatives (e.g. lactulose).[2]
- Grapefruit juice can inhibit the hepatic clearance of amiodarone, resulting in an increase in amiodarone plasma concentrations, so patients should be advised to avoid drinking it.[2]
- Patients complaining of blurred vision or those who see coloured halos in dazzling lights[2] should be referred to their optician/ optometrist or GP. Corneal microdeposits are often reversible on treatment discontinuation. In this instance a patient should be referred back to the GP for treatment review.
- Patients taking amiodarone who develop a new or worsening cough or breathlessness should be referred to their GP for respiratory evaluation.[3]

Flecainide

Patients complaining of double or blurred vision should be referred to their optician or GP. Visual disturbances are usually transient and often disappear on continuing treatment or with dosage reduction.[2] Any alteration in vision is for consideration by the GP so the patient should be referred with the appropriate documentation made on the MUR form.

References

1. Joint Formulary Committee. *British National Formulary 57*. London: BMA and RPSGB, 2009.

2. Electronic Medicines Compendium: Cordarone X, Rythmodan and Tambocor. Available at: http://emc.medicines.org.uk (accessed 19 October 2009).

3. Scottish Intercollegiate Guidelines Network. *Cardiac Arrhythmias in Coronary Heart Disease.* SIGN Guideline 94. Edinburgh: SIGN, 2007. Available at: www.sign.ac.uk/pdf/qrgchd.pdf (accessed 19 October 2009).

3
Respiratory conditions

Asthma

Condition

A common disorder in which there is reversible bronchospasm of the bronchial airways, resulting in chest tightness and wheeze.

Treatment options

Inhaled short-acting β_2 agonist, inhaled corticosteroids, inhaled long-acting β_2 agonist (LABA), leukotriene receptor antagonist, theophylline and oral corticosteroids.[1]

MUR tips

Inhaled short-acting β_2 agonists (e.g. salbutamol)

Excessive use of this inhaler can cause cramp, nervousness and tremor. Patients get instant relief from this inhaler and often feel that their corticosteroid inhaler does not give the same instant relief.[2] During the MUR it is useful to check how often the patient is using this inhaler, because overuse does not provide adequate disease control and may indicate that an escalation of therapy is needed (Figure 3.1).

Step 1: inhaled short-acting agonist β_2 as required

$\downarrow$

Step 2: add inhaled steroid 200–800–mcg/day (beclometasone or equivalent)

$\downarrow$

Step 3:
1. Add long-acting β_2 agonist (LABA)
2. Assess control of asthma:
– good response: continue LABA
– benefit from LABA but control still inadequate: increase dose of inhaled steroid to 800 mcg/day
– no response: stop LABA and increase dose of inhaled steroid to 800 mcg/day

$\downarrow$

Step 4: consider trials of:
1. Increasing inhaled steroids to 2000 mcg/day
2. Addition of fourth drug e.g. leukotriene receptor antagonist or theophylline

$\downarrow$

Step 5:
• Use daily steroid tablet in lowest dose providing adequate control
• Maintain high dose inhaled steroid at 2000 mcg/day
• Refer for specialist care

Figure 3.1   BTS/SIGN guidelines showing stepwise asthma management in adults.[1]

Inhaled corticosteroids (e.g. beclometasone, fluticasone)

Advise patients to rinse the mouth, gargle with water or brush their teeth after using this inhaler. This reduces the incidence of hoarseness caused by candidiasis of the mouth and throat, especially in patients on higher doses. Patients on high doses of corticosteroids may also benefit from a spacer device in order to minimise occurrence of adverse effects. This can be recommended on the MUR form. Patients should be reminded to clean their inhaler device on a weekly basis by wiping the mouthpiece and cover with a dry cloth or tissue.[3]

Inhaled long-acting β_2 agonists (e.g. salmeterol)

The onset of action is slower than short-acting β_2 agonists.[4] Excessive use of this inhaler can cause cramp, nervousness and tremor. Patients using the pressurised metered dose inhaler should be reminded to clean their inhaler device on a weekly basis by wiping the mouthpiece and cover with a dry cloth or tissue.[3]

Leukotriene receptor antagonists (e.g. montelukast)

These are generally well tolerated, although they may cause headache and abdominal pain.[4] Patients should be reminded that leukotriene receptor antagonists are not suitable for relieving symptoms of acute asthma exacerbations.[5]

Theophylline

This has a narrow therapeutic window. Serum theophylline levels should be checked every 6–12 months unless the patient experiences symptoms suggestive of toxicity, e.g. nausea, vomiting, tremor or palpitations.[5] Patients should be maintained on the same brand of theophylline due to differences in bioavailability among brands.[4] If prescribed generically ask the GP to consider prescribing by proprietary name to resolve this potential problem, documenting this recommendation on the MUR form. Smokers who take theophylline and decide to stop smoking should be aware that theophylline blood levels may increase. A reduction in theophylline dose may be required.[5] The patient should be referred back to the GP and the appropriate documentation made on the MUR form.

Oral corticosteroid (e.g. prednisolone)

Short courses are given in acute asthma exacerbations. Adverse effects are uncommon with infrequent, short courses of oral corticosteroids.[5] Doses should be given as a single dose in the morning, after food, to mimic circadian cortisol production.[4] Soluble prednisolone tablets are available for patients who are unable to take large numbers of tablets or patients who experience difficulties in swallowing.

Additional considerations

- Check that patients understand their treatment management strategy. Patients may require further guidance on when to step up or step down their therapy (Figure 3.1).[1]
- Check how regularly patients are ordering their prescription for inhalers, because frequent repeat prescriptions especially for short-acting β_2-agonist inhaler types may indicate poor asthma control.
- Check the patient's inhaler technique. Patients displaying poor inhaler technique with a pressurised metered dose inhaler may benefit from a Haleraid device, the use of which can be demonstrated during the MUR (Figure 3.2). If patients are unable to use a pressurised metered dose inhaler, consider recommending a switch to a breath-actuated or dry powder inhaler device, to aid effective drug administration. If a suggestion for change is required, ensure that the appropriate documentation is made on the MUR form.
- Order placebo inhaler devices from manufacturers to allow patients to demonstrate their inhaler technique during an MUR.
- If patients are using a combination of inhaled short-acting β_2 agonist and/or inhaled LABA with inhaled corticosteroids then

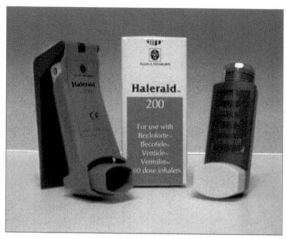

Figure 3.2   Haleraid device.

advise patients to use the β_2-agonist inhaler first and if convenient the inhaled corticosteroid about 15–20 min later.[2]

- Check that patients understand how to use their peak flow meter and that they record their results. Ensure that a peak flow meter is available in the MUR to use as a demonstration aid for patients who require clarification on its use. Encourage patients to maintain a peak flow diary (Figure 3.3). Peak flow diaries are available from organisations such as Asthma UK (visit website – www.asthma.org.uk).

- Advise patients to stop smoking. Signpost to a smoking cessation service.

- Asking patients the following questions will help to determine how well their asthma is controlled:
  - Have you had difficulty sleeping because of your asthma symptoms (including cough)?
  - Have you had your usual symptoms during the day (cough, wheeze, chest tightness or breathlessness)?
  - Has your asthma interfered with your usual activities, e.g. housework, school, work?
  - If patients answer 'yes' to any of these questions then a referral to their asthma nurse may be required, with the appropriate documentation on the MUR form.

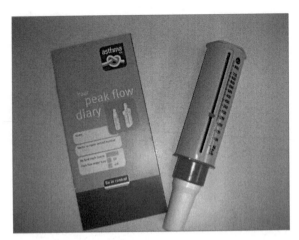

Figure 3.3   Peak flow meter and diary.

References

1. British Thoracic Society and Scottish Intercollegiate Guidelines Network (BTS/SIGN). *British Guidelines on the Management of Asthma*. London: British Thoracic Society, 2008. Available at: www. brit-thoracic.org.uk/Portals/0/Clinical%20Information/Asthma/ Guidelines/asthma_final2008.pdf (accessed 19 October 2009).
2. Melnick P. Patients with asthma: problems revealed by medicines use reviews. *Pharm J* 2008; 280:281.
3. Electronic Medicines Compendium. Clenil and Serevent. Available at: http://emc.medicines.org.uk (accessed 19 October 2009).
4. Joint Formulary Committee. *British National Formulary 57*. London: BMA and RPSGB, 2009.
5. NHS Clinical Knowledge Summaries. Clinical Topic: Asthma. Available at: http://cks.library.nhs.uk/asthma (accessed 19 October 2009).

Chronic obstructive pulmonary disease

Condition

Chronic obstructive pulmonary disease (COPD) is characterised by progressive airflow obstruction, which is not fully reversible. The condition is largely caused by smoking and patients experience a chronic productive cough.

Treatment options

Inhaled short- and long-acting β_2 agonists, inhaled short- and long-acting antimuscarinics, inhaled corticosteroids, oral corticosteroids, aminophylline and theophylline, mucolytics, oxygen therapy, antibiotics and combination therapies.[1]

MUR tips

Inhaled short- and long-acting β_2 agonists (e.g. salbutamol and salmeterol, respectively)

Use of these inhaler types can cause cramp, nervousness and tremor. A rapid onset of bronchodilator action (15–20 min) is seen with short-acting β_2 agonists (e.g. salbutamol and terbutaline).[1] During the MUR explore how often the patient is using these inhaler types because overuse may be an indicator of poor disease control.

Inhaled short- and long-acting antimuscarinics (e.g. ipratropium and tiotropium, respectively)

They have a slower onset of action (after approximately 40 min) compared with short-acting β_2 agonists, so they do not provide instant relief of symptoms.[1,2] Dry mouth is commonly reported with tiotropium.[1,3] Patients can be advised to have a glass of water after taking their inhaler to ease the undesirable effects of a dry mouth. Patients should avoid getting tiotropium powder in their eyes because it can precipitate or worsen narrow-angle glaucoma.[3]

Inhaled corticosteroids (e.g. beclometasone, fluticasone)

Advise patients to rinse their mouth or gargle with water or brush their teeth after using this inhaler. This reduces the incidence of hoarseness caused by candidiasis of the mouth and throat, especially in patients on higher doses. Patients should be reminded to clean their inhaler device on a weekly basis by wiping the mouthpiece and cover with a dry cloth or tissue.[3] Patients on high doses of corticosteroids may also benefit from a spacer device to minimise adverse effects. This can be a recommendation on the MUR form.

Oral corticosteroids (e.g. prednisolone)

Short courses are given in acute COPD exacerbations. Adverse effects are uncommon with infrequent, short courses of oral corticosteroids.[1] Doses should be given as a single dose in the morning, after food, to mimic circadian cortisol production.[2] Soluble prednisolone tablets are available for patients unable to take large numbers of tablets or patients who experience difficulties in swallowing.

Aminophylline/Theophylline

These are considered after a trial of short- and long-acting bronchodilators.[4] Both have a narrow therapeutic window of effect. Symptoms suggestive of toxicity, e.g. nausea, vomiting, tremor or palpitations, must be explored and, if suspected, the patient should be referred to his or her GP. Patients should be maintained on the same brand of theophylline due to differences in bioavailability among brands.[2] If prescribed generically ask the GP to consider prescribing by proprietary name to resolve this potential problem, documenting the recommendation on the MUR form. Smokers who take theophylline and decide to stop smoking should be aware that theophylline blood levels may increase. A reduction in theophylline dose may be required.[1] The patient should be referred back to the GP and the appropriate documentation made on the MUR form.

Mucolytics

Carbocisteine and mecysteine are possible options for people with chronic productive cough.[1,4] A 4-week trial can be initiated and continued if there is improvement in symptoms.[2]

Oxygen therapy

This is considered for patients with respiratory failure.[4] Patients using oxygen therapy must not smoke or use oxygen near to gas stoves or fireplaces because of the fire hazard.[1]

Antibiotics

Amoxicillin, co-amoxiclav, doxycycline, clarithromycin and erythromycin can be prescribed during acute exacerbations of COPD.[1]

Combination therapies

Effective combinations that can increase clinical benefit are:

- β_2 Agonist + anticholinergic
- β_2 Agonist + theophylline
- Anticholinergic + theophylline
- Long-acting β_2 agonist + inhaled corticosteroid.[4]

Additional considerations

- Order placebo inhaler devices from manufacturers to allow patients to demonstrate their inhaler technique during an MUR. Some patients may find it useful to have a demonstration of the Spiriva HandiHaler due to the distinct difference from the other inhaler types available. Ensure that you have a placebo device available. It is worthwhile reminding patients to clean their Spiriva HandiHaler device on a monthly basis.[3]
- Patients can often have the Spiriva HandiHaler device plus capsules on their repeat prescription when they require only the refill capsules. Recommend on the MUR form that the repeat prescription be altered to avoid the patient unnecessarily stock piling the device.
- Advise patients to stop smoking. Signpost to a smoking cessation service.[4]
- Encourage patients to have the annual influenza and pneumococcal immunisation.[4]
- Some patients may have anxiety or depression.[4] Be alert to any signs and symptoms of this and refer the patient appropriately.
- Some patients may be given antibiotics to use during exacerbations of COPD. Check that the patient understands that the antibiotic must be used when sputum is more purulent than usual.[1]

References

1. NHS Clinical Knowledge Summaries. Clinical Topic: COPD. Available at: http://cks.library.nhs.uk/chronic_obstructive_pulmonary_disease (accessed 19 October 2009).
2. Joint Formulary Committee. *British National Formulary 57.* London: BMA and RPSGB, 2009.
3. Electronic Medicines Compendium. Spiriva and Clenil. Available at: http://emc.medicines.org.uk (accessed 19 October 2009).
4. National Institute for Clinical Excellence. *Chronic Obstructive Pulmonary Disease: Management of chronic obstructive pulmonary disease in adults in primary and secondary care: A quick reference guide.* NICE Guideline CG 12. London: NICE, 2004. Available at: www.nice.org.uk/nicemedia/pdf/CG012quickrefguide.pdf (accessed 19 October 2009).

4
Neurological conditions
Alzheimer's disease

Condition

Alzheimer's disease is a common form of dementia which involves loss of mental abilities such as memory.

Treatment options

Acetylcholinesterase inhibitors, e.g. donepezil, galantamine, rivastigmine and memantine.[1]

MUR tips

Donepezil

Used in mild to moderately severe Alzheimer's disease.[1] The dose is often taken in the evening before sleeping. Check whether the patient experiences adverse effects including diarrhoea, muscle cramps, fatigue, nausea, vomiting and insomnia.[2]

Galantamine

Used in mild to moderately severe Alzheimer's disease.[1] The dosage regimen is taken twice daily. Galantamine is associated with weight loss[2] so it is advisable to monitor the patient's weight. Patients can be invited to have their weight monitored at the pharmacy. Check whether the patient experiences any adverse effects of nausea, vomiting, diarrhoea, dyspepsia, headache, dizziness, fatigue, insomnia or confusion.[2]

Rivastigmine

Used in mild to moderately severe Alzheimer's disease.[1] The dosage regimen is taken twice daily. Rivastigmine can cause weight loss so patients should have their weight monitored during therapy.[2] Patients can be invited to have their weight monitored at the pharmacy. Check whether the patient experiences any other adverse effects such as nausea and vomiting.[2]

Memantine

Used in moderately severe to severe Alzheimer's disease.[1] The dosage regimen is once daily. Check whether the patient experiences any adverse effects such as dizziness, somnolence, headache and constipation.[2]

Additional considerations

- Patients who continue to take donepezil, galantamine or rivastigmine should have a medical review every 6 months. The review will include assessment of their Mini-Mental State Examination (MMSE) in addition to functional and behavioural assessment.[3]
- Patients who experience nausea and vomiting on initiation of their treatment can be recommended a suitable over-the-counter

(OTC) preparation. This can help to alleviate these short-lived symptoms. Patients should also be advised to maintain adequate fluid intake.[2]

- Dyspepsia is a common side effect of acetylcholinesterase inhibitors.[2] A suitable OTC preparation can be recommended in these cases, provided that it does not interact with other medications that the patients may be taking. Patients should be advised against using NSAIDs as this will lead to worsening of dyspepsia symptoms.

- Liquid forms of galantamine, rivastigmine and memantine are available for patients who have swallowing difficulties.[2]

References

1. National Institute for Health and Clinical Excellence. *Alzheimer's Disease – donepezil, galantamine, rivastigimne, and memantine.* NICE Guidance TA111. London: NICE, 2007. Available at: www.nice. org.uk/nicemedia/pdf/TA111fullversionamendedSept07.pdf (accessed 19 October 2009).

2. Electronic Medicines Compendium. Aricept, Reminyl, Exelon and Exiba. Available at: http://emc.medicines.org.uk/ (accessed 19 October 2009).

3. NHS Clinical Knowledge Summaries. Clinical Topic: Alzheimer's Disease – Drug Treatments. Available at: http://cks.library.nhs.uk/ alzheimers_drug_treatments/management#171370001 (accessed 19 October 2009).

Parkinson's disease

Condition

Parkinson's disease is a progressive neurodegenerative condition that is caused by the loss of the dopamine-containing cells of the substantia nigra.

Treatment options

Levodopa, dopamine agonists, catechol-O-methyltransferase (COMT) inhibitors, monoamine oxidase B (MAO-B) inhibitors and amantadine (see website – www.parkinsons.org.uk).

MUR tips

Levodopa

Levodopa combined with benserazide forms co-beneldopa (Madopar) or with carbidopa forms co-careldopa (Sinemet). Benserazide and carbidopa prevent the conversion of levodopa to dopamine before it reaches the brain (see www. parkinsons.org.uk). Co-beneldopa can cause nausea, anorexia, vomiting and diarrhoea in the early stages of treatment. Affected patients can be advised to drink fluids while taking their dose because this minimises the adverse effects experienced. Co-careldopa can cause vomiting, diarrhoea and dizziness. Both preparations can cause excessive daytime somnolence.[1] Long-term treatment with levodopa can cause motor fluctuations (on–off phenomenon and dose wearing off) and dyskinesias.[2]

Dopamine agonists

Examples include ropinirole (Requip), rotigotine (Neupro) and cabergoline (Cabaser, Dostinex). These may be used alone or in combination with levodopa. The effects of dopamine agonists last longer than levodopa and are used to reduce both the 'off time' of the condition and levodopa dose required, which results in improvement in motor impairment (see www.parkinsons.org.uk). Common adverse effects include nausea, dyspepsia and somnolence.[1] Ergot-derived dopamine agonists can cause pulmonary and pericardial fibrotic reactions. Patients should be monitored for persistent cough, chest pain, and abdominal pain or tenderness.[3] Caution should be exercised if patients presenting with any of these symptoms request an OTC product.

COMT inhibitors, e.g. entacapone (Comtess)

These should be given with each dose of co-beneldopa or co-careldopa, and act to prolong the action of levodopa in the latter preparations (see website – www.parkinsons.org.uk). Due to its mode of action it can increase the adverse effects caused by levodopa, notably dyskinesias, nausea and vomiting.[2] Entacapone can discolour urine to a reddish-brown colour,[1] so patients can be reassured that this can be expected.

MAO-B inhibitors, e.g. selegiline (Eldepryl and Zelapar)

These can potentiate the side effects caused by levodopa.[1] Selegiline can cause a drop in blood pressure when given on its own. Selegiline is also a mild stimulant, so if prescribed as a once-daily dose it is better taken in the morning rather than at night in order to prevent interference with sleep.[1]

Amantadine (Symmetrel)

This is available in capsule or syrup form. The action of amantadine is weak and short-lived but may be helpful with reducing drug-induced dyskinesias without worsening of parkinsonian symptoms.[2] Patients using amantadine on a long-term basis may develop ankle swelling (see www.parkinsons.org.uk).

Additional considerations

Levodopa

Co-beneldopa is available as a dispersible preparation and is a useful preparation to be taken on wakening to allow the patient to dress. The dispersible tablets should be dispersed in a glass of cold water or squash.[1] Patients who have end-of-dose issues may require a modified-release preparation and should be referred to their GP.

Dopamine agonists

Rotigotine (Neupro) is available as a patch which is applied once daily and may be more suitable for patients with swallowing difficulties.

MAO-B inhibitors

An orodispersible preparation of selegiline (Zelapar) is available which is placed on the tongue and dissolves within 10 s. The patient should be advised not to eat or drink for 5 min after taking the orodispersible tablet in order to allow the selegiline to be absorbed.[1]

- Advise any patient who experiences sudden onset of sleep with any of their medications to avoid driving.[4]
- Advise patients with sleep disturbances to adopt good sleep hygiene measures to minimise this.[4] Advise patients to adopt measures such as increasing day-time activities, ensuring regular sleep hours and relaxation before bedtime (see www.parkinsons.org.uk).

References

1. Electronic Medicines Compendium. Madopar, Sinemet, Cabaser, Neupro, Comtess, Eldepryl, Zelapar. Available at: http://emc.medicines.org.uk (accessed 19 October 2009).
2. NHS Clinical Knowledge Summaries Clinical Topic: Parkinson's Disease. Available at: http://cks.library.nhs.uk/parkinsons_disease (accessed 19 October 2009).
3. Joint Formulary Committee. *British National Formulary 57*. London: BMA and RPSGB, 2009.
4. National Institute for Health and Clinical Excellence. *Parkinson's Disease: Diagnosis and Management in Primary and Secondary Care: A quick reference guide*. NICE Guideline CG 35. London: NICE, 2006. Available at: www.nice.org.uk/nicemedia/pdf/cg035quickrefguide.pdf (accessed 19 October 2009).

Depression

Condition

Depression is a condition of persistent low mood or sadness. It may interfere with sleep and lower self-confidence.

Treatment options

Selective serotonin reuptake inhibitors (SSRIs), tricyclic antidepressants (TCAs), serotonin and noradrenaline reuptake inhibitors (SNRIs), noradrenaline reuptake inhibitors (NRIs), monoamine oxidase inhibitors (MAOIs), mirtazapine and St John's wort.[1]

MUR tips

SSRIs

Examples include citalopram, fluoxetine, paroxetine and sertraline. Citalopram and fluoxetine are prescribed as first-choice antidepressants in moderate-to-severe depression as they are associated with fewer side effects.[2,3] Sertraline is used in patients who have recently had a myocardial infarction or unstable angina. Several cases of extrapyramidal symptoms with paroxetine have been reported to the Medicines and Healthcare products Regulatory Agency (MHRA), formerly known as the Committee on Safety of Medicines (CSM).

SSRIs are commonly associated with nausea, diarrhoea and dyspepsia. Patients should also be monitored for suicidal ideas, increased anxiety or agitation in the early stages of SSRI treatment.[2] These symptoms should prompt immediate referral to the GP. Check that the patient is compliant, because non-compliance may result in treatment failure.

TCAs

Examples include amitriptyline, trazodone, dosulepin and lofepramine. Doses are titrated slowly with TCAs to minimise the risk of adverse effects. TCAs can cause anticholinergic side effects such as dry mouth, blurred vision, constipation and sweating. They should be prescribed in limited quantities because their cardiovascular effects are dangerous in overdose.[1] Lofepramine has fewer anticholinergic side effects and lacks cardiotoxicity problems in overdose.[2,3] Trazodone has no anticholinergic side effects but is very sedating.[2] Check the patient's compliance and explore any possible adverse effects that he or she may be experiencing.

SNRIs

Examples include venlafaxine and duloxetine. Both are used in cases of severe depression.[1] Venlafaxine is associated with nausea, hypertension, dry mouth and insomnia. Its use requires regular blood pressure monitoring,[3] which can be offered during the MUR.

Noradrenaline reuptake inhibitors, e.g. reboxetine

There is a relative lack of data on side effects so careful monitoring is required if a patient is on this therapy.[3] Any adverse events experienced by patients should be reported to the MHRA.

MAOIs, e.g. tranylcypromine and moclobemide

Ensure that patients are aware of the food interactions with MAOIs. Patients on MAOIs should be advised not to eat any tyramine-rich foods such as mature cheese, meat or yeast extracts (e.g. Bovril or Marmite), or pickled herrings because these may cause a dangerous rise in blood pressure.[1]

Mirtazapine

This has few anticholinergic effects but can cause sedation when treatment is initiated.[1] Mirtazapine can cause weight gain so patients should have their weight monitored regularly. This can be done at the pharmacy. It also has the potential to cause agranulocytosis so patients should be advised to report any symptoms of fever, sore throat or signs of infection.[2] The presence of any of these symptoms should prompt immediate referral to the GP.

St John's wort

It may be beneficial in mild-to-moderate depression. Patients should be advised on the variations in the nature and potency of the preparations available and the potential serious interactions with drugs such as oral contraceptives, anticoagulants and anticonvulsants.[3]

Additional considerations

- SSRIs and TCAs can cause hyponatraemia which is more common in elderly people or those taking diuretics. If a patient develops confusion or drowsiness while taking an SSRI or TCA then hyponatraemia should be suspected.[1] In this instance the patient should be referred to the GP.
- Antidepressants often take 4–6 weeks to exert their full effect.[1] Patients should be encouraged to persist with treatment in the early

stages of treatment. Non-compliance with treatment will probably result in treatment failure. It is important to advise patients not to stop taking their antidepressant when their symptoms start to improve because this may result in relapse of their symptoms.

- Antidepressants should be used in therapeutic doses to exert their effects (Table 4.1).[2] Check that the patient is prescribed an appropriate dose for depression.
- Patients with moderate-to-severe depression should continue with antidepressant treatment for 6 months after remission.[3]
- Patients wanting to stop their antidepressant therapy should be informed of the possibility of withdrawal symptoms especially if treatment is stopped abruptly. Doses are often tapered over a 4-week period with some patients requiring longer periods. Fluoxetine can usually be stopped over a shorter period of time.[3] Patients should be reminded to consult their GP to discuss the discontinuation of antidepressant treatment.
- Patients with mild depression who do not want pharmacological treatment may benefit from a structured exercise programme consisting of three (45 min to 1 hour) sessions per week for between 10 and 12 weeks.[3]

Table 4.1 The minimum effective dose and maximum recommended daily dose that should be used for the respective antidepressants[2]

Antidepressant	Usual minimum effective daily dose (mg)	Maximum recommended daily dose (mg)
Citalopram	20	60
Fluoxetine	20	60
Paroxetine	20	20 (MHRA advises against higher doses)
Sertraline	50	200

Table 4.1 *Continued*

Antidepressant	Usual minimum effective daily dose (mg)	Maximum recommended daily dose (mg)
Tricyclic antidepressants	At least 75 (possibly higher)	150–300
Lofepramine	140	210
Trazodone	150	300
Mirtazapine	30	45
Moclobemide	300	600
Reboxetine	8	12
Venlafaxine	75	375 (only under supervision of specialist mental health medical practitioner)

Reproduced with permission from NHS Clinical Knowledge Summaries Library.
MHRA, Medical Health products Regulatory Authority – formerly the Committee on Safety of Medicines (CSM).

References

1. Joint Formulary Committee. *British National Formulary 57.* London: BMA and RPSGB, 2009.
2. NHS Clinical Knowledge Summaries. Clinical Topic: Depression. Available at: http://cks.library.nhs.uk/depression (accessed 19 October 2009).
3. National Institute for Health and Clinical Excellence. *Depression: Management of Depression in Primary and Secondary Care: A quick reference guide.* NICE Guideline CG 23. London: NICE, 2007. Available at: www.nice.org.uk/nicemedia/pdf/CG23quickrefguideamended. pdf (accessed 19 October 2009).

Bipolar disorder

Condition

This is a major mood disorder characterised by periods of elevated mood and periods of severe depression.

Treatment options

Antipsychotics, lithium and semisodium valproate.[1]

MUR tips

Antipsychotics

Examples include risperidone, olanzapine and quetiapine. Weight gain is an adverse effect associated with antipsychotics and patients should have their weight monitored regularly. This can be done at the pharmacy. Antipsychotics can also cause hyperglycaemia and precipitate diabetes so regular blood glucose checks must be carried out.[1] This service can also be offered at the pharmacy.

Lithium

Lithium carbonate is available as tablet formulations of Camcolit, Liskonum and Priadel. Lithium citrate is available as liquid formulations of Priadel and Li-Liquid. (Lithium carbonate 200 mg is equivalent to lithium citrate 509 mg.) Lithium formulations vary in their bioavailability so it is important that prescriptions for lithium are always by brand name.[2] If prescribed generically ask the GP to consider prescribing by proprietary name and document this recommendation on the MUR form. Lithium has a narrow therapeutic window and blood levels are often checked every 3 months in patients who are stable on treatment.[1] Renal and thyroid function tests should also be carried out periodically[1,3] so it is worthwhile checking that the patient attends blood test appointments at their GP surgery.

Semisodium valproate

This is available as Depakote. Adverse effects may include blood disorders so patients should be encouraged to report any signs of bleeding, bruising or sore throat.[3] In this instance a patient should be referred back to the GP immediately. Weight gain is a common adverse effect[3] and patients should have their weight monitored regularly. This can be done at the pharmacy.

Additional considerations

Lithium

Check that patients carry a 'lithium card' and if they do not possess one then issue one from the pharmacy. Lithium cards are obtainable from the National Pharmacy Association (NPA).[2]

- Patients should be advised on how to recognise symptoms of toxicity. These include diarrhoea, vomiting, muscle weakness and lethargy.[2] If a patient experiences any of these adverse effects he or she should be referred to the GP.

- Lithium toxicity can arise from either dehydration or interacting medications. Episodes of dehydration can arise from bouts of diarrhoea and vomiting, and excessive sweating, e.g. after exercise, or from fever associated with infection.[1] Patients should be advised to increase their fluid intake to alleviate the dehydration and consult their GP immediately if symptoms of toxicity are present.
- OTC medicines such as NSAIDs (e.g. ibuprofen) can increase lithium levels whereas indigestion remedies containing sodium bicarbonate can decrease them.[3] It is useful to inform patients of this, because these products can be purchased from non-pharmacy outlets where the expertise on drug interactions is not available.
- Patients who miss a dose(s) should be advised not to account for the missed dose by taking an extra one.[1] Instead they should take their next dose at the time that it is due.
- Non-compliance with therapy can lead to relapse of symptoms.[1] It is important to explore any issues of non-compliance and attempt to resolve them.

Semisodium valproate

Depakote is licensed for treatment of acute mania but sodium valproate (Epilim) is not.[1] It is important to ensure that patients are prescribed the correct product.

References

1. NHS Clinical Knowledge Summaries. Clinical Topic: Bipolar Disorder. Available at: http://cks.library.nhs.uk/bipolar_disorder (accessed 19 October 2009).
2. Joint Formulary Committee. *British National Formulary 57*. London: BMA and RPSGB, 2009.
3. Electronic Medicines Compendium Camcolit, Priadel and Depakote. Available at: http://emc.medicines.org.uk (accessed 19 October 2009).

Schizophrenia

Condition

Schizophrenia is a mental illness where the patient can hallucinate as well as have thought disorders with unusual beliefs.

Treatment options

Atypical antipsychotics and typical antipsychotics.[1]

MUR tips

Atypical antipsychotics

Examples include amisulpride, olanzapine, quetiapine and risperidone. These are recommended as first-choice agents in patients with newly diagnosed schizophrenia.[1] When treatment is started the doses used are at the lower end of the dose range. The full antipsychotic effect develops over several weeks.[2] Patients may experience adverse effects of sedation, weight gain, hyperprolactinaemia, extrapyramidal effects such as abnormal movements of the face or body, and anticholinergic symptoms of dry mouth or blurred vision.[2] Non-compliance due to adverse effects can lead to treatment failure so it is important to explore this thoroughly during the MUR.

Typical antipsychotics

Examples include chlorpromazine, flupentixol, haloperidol and trifluoperazine. Dosage should be in the range 300–1000 mg chlorpromazine equivalents per day[2] (Table 4.2). Typical antipsychotics are associated with more adverse effects than atypical antipsychotics. If a patient is experiencing intolerable adverse effects with a typical antipsychotic then switching to an atypical antipsychotic should be considered.[2] In this instance a patient should be referred to the GP.

Table 4.2 The equivalent doses of oral antipsychotics[3]

Antipsychotic drug	Daily dose (mg)
Chlorpromazine	100
Clozapine	50
Haloperidol	2–3
Pimozide	2
Risperidone	0.5–1.0
Sulpiride	200
Trifluoperazine	5

Reproduced from the BNF. The reader is reminded that the BNF is constantly revised, so for the latest guidelines please consult the current edition of the BNF.

Additional considerations

- Patients taking higher doses of chlorpromazine should be advised of the possibility of developing photosensitivity and the importance of avoiding exposure to direct sunlight.[4]
- Patients on antipsychotics can be offered a weight-monitoring service in the pharmacy if they have concerns about weight gain.
- Atypical antipsychotics can precipitate diabetes[1] so concerned patients can be offered a blood glucose monitoring service in the pharmacy and appropriate referral if test results are abnormal.
- Depot injections are available for patients who are non-compliant with oral treatment or who have a preference for this route of administration.[1] Non-compliant patients should be referred to their GP for a treatment review.
- Antipsychotics are continued for a period of 1–2 years from the start of recovery to prevent any relapses. Patients should not stop antipsychotics suddenly because withdrawal symptoms may develop. Doses are often tapered down over a period of at least 3 weeks.[2] Any patient wanting to stop antipsychotic treatment should discuss this with his or her GP.

References

1. National Institute for Health and Clinical Excellence. *Schizophrenia: Core interventions in the treatment and management of schizophrenia in primary and secondary care.* NICE Guideline CG 82. London: NICE, 2009. Available at: www.nice.org.uk/nicemedia/pdf/CG82FullGuideline.pdf (accessed 19 October 2009).
2. NHS Clinical Knowledge Summaries. Clinical Topic: Schizophrenia. Available at: http://cks.library.nhs.uk/schizophrenia (accessed 19 October 2009).
3. Joint Formulary Committee. *British National Formulary 57.* London: BMA and RPSGB, 2009.
4. Electronic Medicines Compendium. Largactil. Available at: http://emc.medicines.org.uk/ (accessed 19 October 2009).

Epilepsy

Condition

Epilepsy is a condition of recurrent unprovoked seizures. Seizures can be either generalised or partial.

Treatment options

Antiepileptic drugs (AEDs).

MUR tips

Table 4.3 shows the AEDs used according to seizure type.[1]

Table 4.3 Antiepileptic drugs used according to seizure type[1]

Seizure type	First-line drugs	Second-line drugs	Other drugs that may be considered	Drugs to be avoided (may worsen seizures)
Generalised tonic–clonic	Carbamazepine[a] Lamotrigine[b] Sodium valproate Topiramate[a,b]	Clobazam Levetiracetam Oxcarbazepine[a]	Acetazolamide Clonazepam Phenobarbital[a] Phenytoin[a] Primidone[a,c]	Tiagabine Vigabatrin
Absence	Ethosuximide Lamotrigine[b] Sodium valproate	Clobazam Clonazepam Topiramate[a]		Carbamazepine[a] Gabapentin Oxcarbazepine[a] Tiagabine Vigabatrin

[a] Hepatic enzyme-inducing antiepileptic drug.
[b] Should be used as a first choice under circumstances outlined in the NICE technology appraisal TA 76.
[c] Should rarely be initiated – if a barbiturate is required, Phenobarbital is preferred.

Table 4.3 *Continued*

Seizure type	First-line drugs	Second-line drugs	Other drugs that may be considered	Drugs to be avoided (may worsen seizures)
Myoclonic	Sodium valproate	Clobazam Clonazepam Lamotrigine Levetiracetam Piracetam Topiramate[a]		Carbamazepine[c] Gabapentin Oxcarbazepine[a] Tiagabine Vigabatrin
Tonic	Lamotrigine[b] Sodium valproate	Clobazam Clonazepam Levetiracetam Topiramate[a]	Acetazolamide Phenobarbital[a] Phenytoin[a] Primidone[a,c]	Carbamazepine[c] Oxcarbazepine[a]
Atonic	Lamotrigine[b] Sodium valproate	Clobazam Clonazepam Levetiracetam Topiramate[a]	Acetazolamide Phenobarbital[a] Primidone[a,c]	Carbamazepine[c] Oxcarbazepine[a] Phenytoin[a]
Focal with/without secondary generalisation	Carbamazepine[a] Lamotrigine[b] Oxcarbazepine[a,b] Sodium valproate Topiramate[a,b]	Clobazam Gabapentin Levetiracetam Phenytoin[a] Tiagabine	Acetazolamide Clonazepam Phenobarbital[a] Primidone[a,c]	

[a] Hepatic enzyme-inducing antiepileptic drug.
[b] Should be used as a first choice under circumstances outlined in the NICE technology appraisal TA 76.
[c] Should rarely be initiated – if a barbiturate is required, Phenobarbital is preferred.
Reproduced with permission from NICE.

Acetazolamide

This commonly causes nausea, vomiting and diarrhoea.[1]

Carbamazepine

This is a liver-inducing AED so it can increase metabolism of concomitantly administered drugs such as the oral contraceptive. This reduces the contraceptive's effectiveness. Common adverse effects experienced on initiation of treatment are allergic skin reactions and blurred vision.[1,2]

Clobazam

This can commonly cause drowsiness and confusion. Tolerance may develop with long-term use.[1,2]

Clonazepam

This can cause drowsiness and fatigue which usually disappear as treatment continues.[1,2]

Ethosuximide

This can cause nausea, headache and drowsiness on initiation of treatment.[1,2]

Gabapentin

This commonly causes drowsiness, fatigue and dizziness.[1,2]

Lamotrigine

Common adverse effects include headache, tiredness, rash, nausea, dizziness and insomnia.[1,2] Lamotrigine can reduce the effectiveness of the combined oral contraceptive.[2]

Levetiracetam

Adverse effects that most commonly occur in the first month of treatment include dizziness and drowsiness.[1,2]

Oxcarbazepine

This is an analogue of carbamazepine so it also induces liver enzymes. Oxcarbazepine can reduce the effectiveness of oral contraceptives. Common adverse effects include headache, diplopia and nausea.[1,2]

Phenobarbital

This is a liver enzyme-inducing AED so it can reduce the effectiveness of oral contraceptives and warfarin. Common adverse effects include drowsiness, lethargy and mental depression.[1,2]

Phenytoin

This is a liver enzyme-inducing AED and can reduce the effectiveness of oral contraceptives. Common adverse effects include skin rash, drowsiness, ataxia and slurred speech.[1,2] Phenytoin has a narrow therapeutic range.[3]

Piracetam

This can cause insomnia, drowsiness and depression. Weight gain is associated with piracetam[1,2] and patients can be offered a weight-monitoring service in the pharmacy.

Primidone

This is a liver enzyme-inducing AED and can reduce the effectiveness of oral contraceptives. It can commonly cause drowsiness and listlessness especially at the start of treatment.[1,2]

Sodium valproate

This can cause weight gain due to increased appetite, which is usually seen after 3 months of treatment.[2] Patients can be invited for a weight-monitoring service at the pharmacy if they have concerns about this. Other adverse effects include transient hair loss, tremor at higher doses and menstrual irregularities in adolescent girls.[2] Epilim tablets are hygroscopic, so, during the MUR, check that the patient is not removing the tablets from the foil until immediately before they are taken.[4]

Tiagabine

This causes dizziness, tiredness and concentration difficulties.[1,2]

Topiramate

This is a weak liver enzyme-inducing AED so it can reduce the effectiveness of oral contraceptives. Common adverse effects include drowsiness, headache and dizziness.[1,2]

Vigabatrin

Commonly causes drowsiness, nausea, agitation and depression. Visual field defects can occur in one-third of patients and can develop at any time during treatment with vigabatrin. Check that patients are having visual field tests at 6-monthly intervals.[1,2]

Additional considerations

• Non-compliance with medication may result in seizures. If a patient is non-compliant due to inability to swallow the tablet or capsule formulation prescribed, an alternative may be recommended on the MUR form for consideration by the prescriber. Bioavailability variations exist between dosage forms that must be considered when alternative forms are recommended (Table 4.4).

- Some AEDs interact with the contraceptive pill. It is important to ensure that the patient is using adequate contraceptive measures.
- Driving: AEDs can cause drowsiness, which may affect a patient's ability to drive.
- Patients who have been seizure free for a period of 2 years may ask about stopping treatment. This should be done under the guidance of a specialist[2] so refer the patient to the GP. The Driving and Vehicle Licensing Agency (DVLA) recommend patients not to drive during the period of AED withdrawal and for a period of 6 months afterwards. [2]

Table 4.4 Alternative formulations available for some antiepileptic drugs (AEDs)[4]

AED	Alternative formulations available for patients who are unable to swallow tablet or capsule preparations
Carbamazepine	Chewable tablets and liquid
Ethosuximide	Syrup
Lamotrigine	Dispersible tablets
Levetiracetam	Oral solution
Oxcarbazepine	Suspension
Phenytoin	Suspension

Table 4.4 *Continued*

AED	Alternative formulations available for patients who are unable to swallow tablet or capsule preparations
Sodium valproate	Crushable tablets, syrup and modified-release granule sachet
Topiramate	Topamax sprinkle capsules. The contents of the capsule can be sprinkled on soft foods such as yoghurt
Vigabatrin	Powder sachet

References

1. National Institute for Clinical Excellence. *Epilepsy in Adults: The Epilepsies: Diagnosis and management of epilepsies in adults in primary and secondary care: A quick reference guide.* NICE Guideline CG 20. London: NICE, 2004. Available at: www.nice.org.uk/nicemedia/pdf/CG020adultsquickrefguide.pdf (accessed 19 October 2009).
2. NHS Clinical Knowledge Summaries. Clinical Topic: Epilepsy. Available at: http://cks.library.nhs.uk/epilepsy (accessed 19 October 2009).
3. Joint Formulary Committee. *British National Formulary 57.* London: BMA and RPSGB, 2009.
4. Electronic Medicines Compendium Tegretol, Zarontin, Lamictal, Keppra, Trileptal, Epanutin, Topamax Sprinkle and Sabril. Available at: http://emc.medicines.org.uk/ (accessed 19 October 2009).

Anxiety disorders

Condition

A condition that may consist of loss of mood and changes in appetite, weight and sleep patterns. Panic attacks may also be present.

Treatment options

Benzodiazepines, SSRIs, TCAs and buspirone.[1]

MUR tips

Benzodiazepines

Examples include chlordiazepoxide, diazepam, oxazepam and lorazepam. Benzodiazepines are often prescribed as a short course of treatment in order to avoid dependency.[1] Common adverse effects include drowsiness and sedation.[3]

SSRIs such as paroxetine

These are used for long-term management of anxiety disorders.[2] Common adverse effects associated with use include nausea, vomiting and diarrhoea. Patients should be reassured that these adverse effects usually subside with the treatment course.[1]

TCAs

The most commonly used TCAs are clomipramine and imipramine.[2] TCAs are considered if SSRIs are unsuitable or there is no improvement in the condition. They can also be used for long-term management of anxiety disorders.[2] Common adverse effects associated with use include anticholinergic effects such as dry mouth, sedation and constipation.

Buspirone

This is often used as a short-term treatment option. It is well tolerated and associated with a low risk of dependence and withdrawal problems.[1] Common adverse effects associated with use include headache and dizziness.[3]

Additional considerations

- Patients who are prescribed an SSRI or TCA should be informed of a potential increase in anxiety symptoms on initiation of treatment. Patients should also be informed of the possibility of withdrawal symptoms if treatment is stopped abruptly or if doses are missed.[2]
- Patients can be signposted to anxiety support groups if available.[2]
- Exercise routines are beneficial for patients with anxiety disorders.[2] Patients can be offered general advice about exercise that can be undertaken.

References

1. GP Notebook. Anxiety Available at: www.gpnotebook.co.uk/simplepage.cfm?ID= 1778778113 (accessed 19 October 2009).
2. National Institute for Health and Clinical Excellence. *Anxiety: Management of anxiety (panic disorder, with or without agoraphobia,*

and generalised anxiety disorder) in adults in primary, secondary and community care. A quick reference guide. NICE Guideline CG 22. London: NICE, 2007. Available at: www.nice.org.uk/nicemedia/ pdf/CG022quickrefguideamended.pdf (accessed 19 October 2009).

3. Electronic Medicines Compendium. Librium and Buspar. Available at: http://emc.medicines.org.uk/ (accessed 19 October 2009).

Pain control

Condition

An unpleasant sensation that can occur as a result of injury or disease, with varying severity.

Treatment options

Non-opioid analgesics and opioid analgesics.[1]

MUR tips

Non-opioid analgesics

Examples include paracetamol, NSAIDs and compound analgesics.

Paracetamol

This is the first choice analgesic for patients with mild-to-moderate pain. Paracetamol is a well-tolerated and effective analgesic if used at full therapeutic doses (1g up to four times a day).[2] During the MUR, check that the patient takes paracetamol regularly to achieve maximal benefit from treatment. Patients can often feel that it is an ineffective analgesic especially when taken on an 'as-required' basis and may express a wish for the pharmacist to recommend an alternative analgesic. In this instance it is worthwhile encouraging patients to use paracetamol at the full therapeutic dose before considering an alternative.[2]

NSAIDs

Examples include ibuprofen and diclofenac. Low-dose ibuprofen is the preferred first choice due to its lower risk of gastrointestinal complications.[2] Adverse effects associated with use include gastrointestinal adverse effects, aggravating asthma and renal impairment.[1] If patients experience dyspepsia while taking an NSAID it is advisable to refer them to the GP for consideration of the addition of a gastroprotective agent. This recommendation can be documented on the MUR form. If a patient's pain is uncontrolled by NSAID alone the patient can be advised to use paracetamol at therapeutic doses in addition.[2]

Compound analgesics

Examples include co-codamol and co-dydramol. There is little evidence that low opioid dose compound analgesics have benefits over paracetamol or aspirin alone. The low dose of opioid in the preparation may be enough to cause opioid adverse effects such as constipation.[1,3] During the MUR explore the patient's use of compound analgesics and their perceived effectiveness.

Opioid analgesics

These are classed as weak opioids and strong opioids.

Weak opioids

Examples include codeine and dihydrocodeine. Weak opioids are used for patients who experience an inadequate response to non-opioids.[2] Adverse effects associated with use include nausea, vomiting, constipation and dry mouth.[1] Weak opioids can be used in addition to paracetamol and/or an NSAID.[2] Check whether the patient is experiencing any adverse effects and discuss options available to alleviate the problem.

Strong opioids

Examples include morphine. Adverse effects associated with use include nausea, vomiting, constipation and dry mouth.[1] During the MUR explore previous analgesics that the patient has used and perceived reasons for their ineffectiveness. If a dose increase is required with a strong opioid, it is important to check that the dose increase made is within the recommended range (e.g. for an adult taking either morphine or oxycodone a dose increase should not be 50% higher than the previous dose).[4]

Additional considerations

- Headaches are associated with regular use of analgesics especially combination products. Explore this during the MUR and advise patients with a previous history of headaches to avoid taking analgesics on a daily basis.[3]
- Remind patients who take paracetamol on a regular basis to avoid taking OTC products containing paracetamol, e.g. cold and flu remedies, so as not to exceed the maximum recommended dose.[3]

References

1. Joint Formulary Committee. *British National Formulary 57*. London: BMA and RPSGB, 2009.
2. National Prescribing Centre. The withdrawal of co-proxamol: alternative analgesics for mild to moderate pain. *MeReC Bull*

2006; 16(4):13–16. Available at: www.npc.co.uk/ebt/merec/pain/otherback/resources/merec_bulletin_vol16_no4.pdf (accessed 19 October 2009).

3. National Prescribing Centre. The use of oral analgesics in primary care. *MeReC Bull* 2000; 11(1):1–4. Available at: www.npc.co.uk/ebt/merec/pain/otherback/resources/merec_bulletin_vol11_no1.pdf (accessed 19 October 2009).

4. National Patient Safety Agency (NPSA). *Reducing Dosing Errors with Opioid Medicines*. London: NPSA, 2008. Available at: www.npsa.nhs.uk/nrls/alerts-and-directives/rapidrr/reducing-dosing-errors-with-opioid-medicines/ (accessed 19 October 2009).

Obesity

Condition

Obesity is determined by the individual's body mass index (BMI) (Table 4.5). BMI is worked out by:[1]

BMI = Weight (kg)/Height squared (m^2)

Table 4.5 The classification of overweight or obesity[2]

Classification	BMI (kg/m^2)
Healthy weight	18.5–24.9
Overweight	25–29.9
Obese I	30–34.9
Obese II	35–39.9
Obese III	≥ 40

Reproduced with permission from NICE.

Treatment options

Pharmacological treatments are considered after dietary, exercise and behavioural approaches have been tried.[2] Options include orlistat and sibutramine.[1]

MUR tips

Overweight and obese patients have an increased health risk associated with their weight and waist circumference (Table 4.6). This can be sensitively approached during the MUR.

Orlistat

This is used for obese individuals. Common adverse effects include abdominal discomfort, faecal urgency, oily spotting and fatty stools.[1,3] If a patient is taking a multivitamin supplement he or she is best advised to take it 2 hours after a dose of orlistat. There is a theoretical risk that orlistat can reduce the absorption of the fat-soluble vitamins (A, D, E and K).[1]

Sibutramine

This is used for obese individuals. Adverse effects experienced include insomnia, nausea, dry mouth and constipation.[3] Other adverse effects include an increase in blood pressure and heart rate.[1] A patient can be offered a blood pressure-monitoring service at the pharmacy during treatment with sibutramine. It is recommended that blood pressure be checked every 2 weeks for the first 3 months of treatment, then monthly for the next 3 months, then every 3 months.[1,3]

Note. This product had its licence suspended in January 2010.

Table 4.6 An assessment of health risks associated with overweight and obese adults[2]

BMI classification	Waist circumference		
	Low	High	Very high
Overweight	No increased risk	Increased risk	High risk
Obesity I	Increased risk	High risk	Very high risk

For men, waist circumference of <94 cm is low, 94–102 cm is high and >102 cm is very high.
For women, waist circumference of <80 cm is low, 80–88 cm is high and >88 cm is very high.
Reproduced with permission from NICE.

Additional considerations

- Treatment with either orlistat or sibutramine for longer than 3 months should be considered only if the patient has lost at least 5% of their initial body weight since starting drug treatment.[3]
- Orlistat can be continued beyond a year if its risks and benefits have been discussed with the patient. Sibutramine treatment is recommended for only 1 year.[3] During the MUR, check the length of the treatment period with the patient.
- The MUR is an ideal opportunity to discuss strategies to help patients achieve and maintain a healthy weight (Table 4.7).
- Encourage patients to check their weight periodically.[2] A weight-monitoring service can be offered at the pharmacy to provide the patient with encouragement and support.
- Weight gain may also be related to other medicines that the patient is taking. Again a weight-monitoring service can be offered at the pharmacy.

Table 4.7 Strategies to help patients achieve and maintain a healthy weight[2]

Diet	Exercise
Meals should be based on starchy food such as potatoes, bread, rice and pasta (wholegrain where possible).	Encourage patients to make activities such as swimming, walking, cycling and gardening part of their everyday activities.
Advise patients to eat plenty of fibre-rich foods such as oats, beans, peas, lentils, grains, fruit and vegetables.	Advise patients to minimise periods of sedentary activities such as sitting for long periods of time watching television or playing video games.
Patients should be advised to eat five portions of fruit and vegetables per day.	Advise patients to build activities into the working day such as taking the stairs instead of the lift or going for a walk at lunchtime.
Patients should eat a low-fat diet and avoid increasing fat or calorie intake.	
Fried food, confectionery high in added sugars and other foods high in fat and sugar such as some take-away and fast foods should be eaten as little as possible.	
Encourage patients to eat breakfast.	
Patients should be advised to watch portion sizes of meals and snacks and how often they are eating.	

References

1. NHS Clinical Knowledge Summaries. Clinical Topic: Obesity. Available at: http://cks.library.nhs.uk/obesity (accessed 19 October 2009).
2. National Institute for Health and Clinical Excellence. *Obesity. Guidance on prevention, identification, assessment and management of overweight and obesity in adults and children.* NICE Guideline CG 43. London: NICE, 2006. Available at: www.nice.org.uk/nicemedia/pdf/CG43NICEGuideline.pdf (accessed 19 October 2009).
3. National Prescribing Centre. The drug management of obesity. *MeReC Bull* 2008;18(5):1–8. Available at: www.npc.co.uk/ebt/merec/therap/obes/resources/merec_bulletin_vol18_no5.pdf (accessed 19 October 2009).

5
Endocrine conditions
Type 1 diabetes

Condition

A condition of insulin deficiency.

Treatment options

Insulin injections: short-acting, intermediate-acting, biphasic and long-acting insulins (Table 5.1 and Figure 5.1).[1]

Table 5.1 Examples from each insulin category[1]

Short-acting insulin	Intermediate-acting insulin	Biphasic insulin	Long-acting insulin
Actrapid	Insulatard	NovoMix 30	Levemir
Humulin S	Humulin I	Humalog Mix25 and -50	Lantus
NovoRapid		Mixtard 10/20/30/40/50	Hypurin Bovine Protamine Zinc
Humalog		Humulin M3	

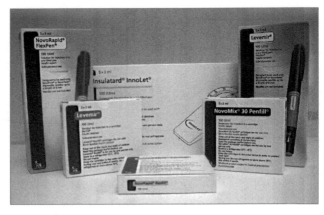

Figure 5.1   Insulin preparations.

MUR tips

Short-acting insulins

They have a fast onset of action and are usually injected 15–30 min before a meal.[1]

Intermediate-acting insulins

The onset of action is approximately 1–2 hours. The dosage regimen is combined with short-acting insulin and administered twice daily.[1]

Biphasic insulins

The onset of action is within 15–30 min, with a maximal effect reached within 1–4 hours. The dosage regimen is usually twice-daily administration with a duration of action of 24 hours.[2]

Long-acting insulins

The dosage regimen is often once-daily administration, although insulin detemir can be given twice daily. Long-acting insulin is used with short-acting insulin.[1]

Additional considerations

- During the MUR check that the patient is adhering to the correct storage requirements of insulin. All insulin cartridges/pens must be refrigerated unless they are in use, in which case they can be kept at room temperature (not above 30°C). Insulin pens/cartridges that are kept at room temperature can be used for a period of 4–6 weeks depending on the insulin brand.[2] Check what reminder systems the patient uses to remember the opening date of the insulin preparation and ensure that the preparation is not being used after the recommended 4–6 weeks.
- Patients should be advised to rotate the injection site to prevent lipodystrophy (fatty lumps that may develop in the skin). Injection sites include the abdominal wall, thigh, and gluteal or deltoid region.[2]
- Order placebo insulin pens and cartridge devices from the manufacturers in order to use as demonstration aids during the MUR. It is worthwhile checking if patients are experiencing any difficulties in using their injecting device. If so, the correct administration can be demonstrated using the placebo device.
- Check that patients know when to adjust their insulin doses, especially during illness, changes of physical activity and in their usual diet, and if transferring to another insulin preparation.[2]
- Patients with inadequate insulin dosage or those who do not take their insulin may experience symptoms of hyperglycaemia. These include thirst, nausea, vomiting, drowsiness, flushed dry skin, dry mouth and loss of appetite, as well as an acetone odour to their breath.[2] Explore and try to resolve any issues with

non-compliance. If a patient is compliant and requires a dose adjustment, refer them to their GP or diabetes nurse, documenting this on the MUR form.

- If the insulin dose is too high patients may have symptoms of hypoglycaemia. Patients should be referred to their GP or diabetes nurse for dose adjustment.
- Patients travelling should be advised on how to transport their insulin (e.g. using Frio insulin cases) and when to administer their dose, taking into account time zone differences. This can be done by keeping a wristwatch set at the time of the country from which they are departing and administering their dose according to their usual time.
- Check that patients are testing their blood glucose appropriately. Check their use and disposal mechanisms for lancets and testing strips.[3]
- For patients who have a blood glucose meter, check that they are calibrating the meter and know how to interpret results.[3] Patients should maintain a blood glucose level of 4–7 mmol/L before meals and <9 mmol/L after meals.[1]
- Encourage patients with uncontrolled diabetes to record their glucose readings in a 'diabetes diary'.[3]
- Check that the patient has his or her HbA1c (glycated haemoglobin) measured every 3–6 months and understands the results. The aim should be to maintain the HbA1c at 6.5%.[1]
- Patients may regularly purchase over-the-counter (OTC) medicines that have a high sugar content.[3] It is worthwhile advising patients on suitable sugar-free alternatives that are available.
- Patients should be encouraged to maintain moderate levels of physical activity (e.g. daily walking) as a life-long lifestyle modification.[4]
- Patients should be encouraged to maintain normal body weight (BMI <25). Invite patients to a pharmacy weight-monitoring service.
- Advise patients to stop smoking. Signpost smokers to a smoking cessation service.[4]
- Patients should also be advised to maintain good foot hygiene and encouraged to see a podiatrist/chiropodist regularly.

References

1. Joint Formulary Committee. *British National Formulary 57.* London: BMA and RPSGB, 2009.
2. Electronic Medicines Compendium. Actrapid, Insulatard and Novomix 30. Available at: http://emc.medicines.org.uk/ (accessed 19 October 2009).
3. Laiglesia N. Patients with diabetes: problems revealed by medicine use reviews. *Pharm J* online 2007; July:PM3. Available at: www.pharmj.com/MedicinesManagement/editorial/200707/features/p03diabetes.htm (accessed 16 November 2009).
4. Scottish Intercollegiate Guidelines Network. *Management of Diabetes, Quick reference guide.* Guideline 55. Edinburgh: SIGN, 2001. Available at: www.sign.ac.uk/pdf/qrg55.pdf (accessed 19 October 2009).

Type 2 diabetes

Condition

Type 2 diabetes is the result of a combination of insulin resistance and pancreatic β-cell failure, which results in insufficient insulin secretion.

Treatment options

Oral hypoglycaemic drugs: metformin, insulin secretagogues (sulphonylureas and meglitinides), thiazolidinediones (glitazones) and insulin.[1]

MUR tips

Metformin

First-choice treatment for overweight patients.[2] Metformin can cause diarrhoea and abdominal pain on initiation of treatment. The frequency and persistence of these symptoms are dose dependent.[1] Advise patients to take metformin after food to minimise these adverse effects.[3] Patients who are unable to tolerate metformin may benefit from a modified-release preparation.[1] In this instance a patient should be referred to the diabetes nurse.

Insulin secretagogues (sulphonylureas and meglitinides)

Sulphonylureas

Gliclazide, glimepiride and glipizide are the sulphonylureas of choice. Glimepiride and glipizide are longer-acting agents.[1] Glibenclamide and chlorpropamide are not recommended for routine use because they are long acting and have a higher risk of hypoglycaemia.[2] Patients who are more prone to hypoglycaemia include elderly people, frail people, those with renal or hepatic impairment and those who have irregular meal times. These patients would benefit from taking gliclazide, glimepiride or glipizide because these agents are less likely to cause hypoglycaemia.[1]

Meglitinides (e.g. nateglinide and repaglinide)

These drugs have a rapid onset and short duration of action. They should be taken 30 min before a meal. Adverse effects associated with use may include abdominal pain, nausea, diarrhoea and constipation.[2]

Thiazolidinediones (e.g. pioglitazone)

These can be used as monotherapy, dual therapy in combination with metformin or triple therapy in combination with metformin and a sulphonylurea. Patients on triple therapy may be at increased risk of hypoglycaemia.[1] Thiazolidinediones can cause visual disturbances so referral to an optician/optometrist is required if patients complain of deterioration in vision.[2]

Insulin

This is initiated if the patient is unable to achieve HbA1c <7.5% while on other glucose-lowering medications.[4] (See previous section for details on insulin preparations.)

Additional considerations

- Sulphonylureas and thiazolidinediones can cause weight gain[2] which may lead to non-compliance. Advise patients to monitor their weight and aim to maintain a normal body weight (BMI <25). Patients can also be invited to have their weight monitored at the pharmacy.
- Advise patients to stop smoking. Signpost smokers to a smoking cessation service.
- Patients should also be advised to maintain good foot hygiene and encouraged to see a podiatrist/chiropodist regularly.
- Offer patients healthy lifestyle and dietary advice, in order to help them achieve and maintain an ideal body weight.
- Other complications of diabetes include hypertension, hyperlipidaemia, renal damage, altered vision, depression and neuropathic complications.[4] Patients are likely to be taking other medicines, so it is important to check their understanding and compliance with concomitant treatments.
- Check that patients who measure their blood glucose levels are testing appropriately. Check their use and disposal mechanisms for lancets and testing strips.[3]
- For patients on insulin who have a blood glucose meter, check that they are calibrating the meter and know how to interpret the results.[3] Patients should aim for a blood glucose level of 4–7 mmol/L before meals and <9 mmol/L after meals.[2]
- Encourage patients with uncontrolled diabetes to record their glucose readings in a 'diabetes diary'.[3]

- Patients experiencing frequent hypoglycaemic episodes should be advised to:
    - have regular meals and avoid missing meals
    - adjust their calorie intake according to any change in their activity levels
    - reduce their alcohol consumption.[1]

References

1. NHS Clinical Knowledge Summaries. Clinical Topic: Type 2 Diabetes. Available at: www.cks.library.nhs.uk/diabetes_type_2 (accessed 19 October 2009).
2. Joint Formulary Committee. *British National Formulary 57*. London: BMA and RPSGB, 2009.
3. Laiglesia N. Patients with diabetes: problems revealed by medicine use reviews. *Pharm J* online 2007; July:PM3. Available at: www. pharmj.com/MedicinesManagement/editorial/200707/features/ p03diabetes.htm (accessed 16 November 2009).
4. National Institute for Health and Clinical Excellence. *Type 2 Diabetes: The management of type 2 diabetes: A quick reference guide*. NICE Guidance CG 66. London: NICE, 2008. Available at: www. nice.org.uk/nicemedia/pdf/CG66T2DQRG.pdf (accessed 19 October 2009).

Hypothyroidism

Condition

A condition of underactive thyroid gland resulting in the underproduction of thyroid hormone.

Treatment options

Levothyroxine and liothyronine.[1]

MUR tips

- Levothyroxine should be taken before breakfast to mimic the body's circadian thyroid hormone release. In adults maintenance doses ranging from 75 mcg to 150 mcg are used.[1] Excessive doses can cause tachycardia, muscle cramps, headache and diarrhoea.[2]
- Levothyroxine has a narrow therapeutic range and small changes in absorption or metabolism can affect thyroid hormone levels.[1] Some drug interactions with levothyroxine include carbamazepine, phenytoin, warfarin and amiodarone.
- Liothyronine has a similar action to levothyroxine but is rapidly metabolised and has a rapid effect. It is used in severe hypothyroid states when a rapid response is desired.[3]

Additional considerations

- Check if patients are taking any other supplements containing calcium or iron. Calcium and iron can reduce the absorption of levothyroxine[1] so patients should be advised to leave a period of 2 hours between taking a supplement and taking levothyroxine.
- Patients who are stable on treatment should have their thyroid-stimulating hormone (TSH) and free thyroxine (T_4) measured annually.[1] Altered blood test results may be an indication of non-compliance with therapy. It is ideal to conduct an MUR if a patient has recently had a dose change, especially if they are unsure why.

References

1. NHS Clinical Knowledge Summaries. Clinical Topic: Hypothyroidism. Available at: http://cks.library.nhs.uk/hypothyroidism (accessed 19 October 2009).
2. Actavis. Summary of product characteristics: Levothyroxine 50 mcg tablets. Available at: www.actavis.co.uk/NR/rdonlyres/ F64FE7FB-1411-4E42-A0CE-8DB1C2B1AD51/0/ Levothyroxine50mcgT6295spc.pdf (accessed 19 October 2009).
3. Joint Formulary Committee. *British National Formulary 57*. London: BMA and RPSGB, 2009.

Hyperthyroidism

Condition

A condition of overactive thyroid gland resulting in the overproduction of thyroid hormones.

Treatment options

Antithyroid drugs, e.g. carbimazole, propylthiouracil and β blockers.[1]

MUR tips

Carbimazole

The initial dose range is 15–40 mg daily with larger doses used occasionally.[1] The maintenance dose range is 5–15 mg daily.[2] Treatment can be given for up to 18 months. Carbimazole is a vitamin K antagonist so it can intensify effects of anticoagulants;[2] therefore ensure that patients taking anticoagulants are aware of this.

Propylthiouracil

Initial doses of 200–400 mg are given. Once a patient is euthyroid the maintenance dose range is 50–150 mg daily.[1] Adverse effects associated with use may include nausea, vomiting and stomach upsets.[2]

β Blockers

Propranolol is the β blocker used most often for symptomatic control of hyperthyroidism. Others that can be used include metoprolol and nadolol. β Blockers can cause coldness of extremities, nausea, fatigue and sleep disturbances.[3]

Additional considerations

- Carbimazole and propylthiouracil can cause agranulocytosis so patients should be warned of the possibility of developing sore throats, bruising, mouth ulcers, fever or malaise.[2,3] It is rare for these symptoms to develop but if presented it is likely to be during the first 3 months of therapy.[3] If any of these symptoms occur, patients should be referred to their GP.
- Carbimazole and propylthiouracil can cause skin rashes in 5% of people. This side effect may resolve spontaneously without stopping treatment.[3]

References

1. Joint Formulary Committee. *British National Formulary 57.* London: BMA and RPSGB, 2009.
2. Electronic Medicines Compendium. Neomercazole and Propylthiouracil. Available at: http://emc.medicines.org.uk (accessed 19 October 2009).
3. NHS Clinical Knowledge Summaries. Clinical Topic: Hyperthyroidism. Available at: http://cks.library.nhs.uk/hyperthyroidism (accessed 19 October 2009).

The menopause and hormone replacement therapy

Condition

The menopause is the time when menstruation stops completely.

Treatment options

Oestrogen-only hormone replacement therapy (HRT), oestrogen combined with progesterone HRT, tibolone and clonidine.[1]

MUR tips

- HRT is given to alleviate menopausal symptoms such as vaginal atrophy or vasomotor symptoms (e.g. flushes or sweats).[2]
- Oestrogen-only HRT is used in women who do not have a uterus. Available preparations include oral tablets (taken daily), transdermal patches (applied once or twice weekly) or gels (applied daily), and vaginal creams or pessaries[1] (Table 5.2).
- Oestrogen combined with progesterone HRT (combined HRT): used in women with an intact uterus. Preparations available include oral tablets (taken daily) and transdermal patches (applied once or twice weekly) (Table 5.2). Progesterone is required in women with an intact uterus

to reduce the risk of endometrial hyperplasia and cancer. Continuous combined HRT may produce irregular bleeding or spotting in the first 4–6 months of treatment.[1]

- Tibolone has oestrogenic, progestogenic and weak androgenic properties. It is used as an alternative to combined HRT in postmenopausal women who wish to have amenorrhoea.[1]
- Clonidine is used to reduce symptoms of the menopause in women who cannot take an oestrogen preparation.[2] Clonidine is associated with side effects of hypotension, dizziness, dry mouth, fluid retention and nausea. It may also aggravate depression or cause insomnia.[1]

Table 5.2 Examples of each type of hormone replacement therapy (HRT)[2]

Oestrogen-only HRT	Oestrogen combined with progesterone HRT
Premarin (oral tablet)	Premique (oral tablet)
Climaval (oral tablet)	Prempak-C (oral tablet)
Elleste-Solo (oral tablet)	Elleste-Duet (oral tablet)
Estraderm MX (transdermal patch)	Estracombi (transdermal patch)
Evorel (transdermal patch)	Evorel (transdermal patch)
Oestrogel (transdermal gel)	Femoston (oral tablet)
Sandrena (transdermal gel)	Kliofem (oral tablet)
Ovestin (vaginal cream)	Kliovance (oral tablet)
Vagifem (vaginal tablet)	Trisequens (oral tablet)

Additional considerations

- Weight gain is common around the time of the menopause. Reassure women that HRT does not cause significant further weight gain.[1]
- HRT can cause fluid retention, bloating, breast tenderness and enlargement, leg cramps and dyspepsia. Encourage women to persist with therapy for 3 months because most adverse effects resolve with increased duration of use. The following are suggestions for alleviating adverse effects associated with HRT:
  - leg cramps can be alleviated by regular exercise and stretching of calf muscles
  - dyspepsia can be minimised by advising women to take their HRT with food
  - breast tenderness may be improved by eating a low-fat and high-carbohydrate diet.[1]
- Encourage all women to adopt healthy lifestyle measures to minimise symptoms of the menopause. These include:
  - taking regular exercise, sleeping in a cooler room and wearing lighter clothes all help to minimise hot flushes and night sweats
  - avoiding spicy foods, caffeine and alcohol also help to minimise hot flushes and night sweats.[1]
- Women wanting to stop HRT should be advised to gradually reduce the dose rather than stop abruptly.[1]
- Women undergoing major surgery should be advised to stop the HRT 4–6 weeks before surgery.[2]
- Advise women who smoke to stop. Signpost to a smoking cessation service.

References

1. NHS Clinical Knowledge Summaries. Clinical Topic: Menopause. Available at: http://cks.library.nhs.uk/menopause (accessed 19 October 2009).
2. Joint Formulary Committee. *British National Formulary 57*. London: BMA and RPSGB, 2009.

Contraception

Condition

Contraception is used to prevent an unwanted pregnancy. Hormonal contraceptives act by preventing ovulation.

Treatment options

Combined oral contraceptives (COCs), progestogen-only pill (POP), combined contraceptive patch, long-acting progestogens and intra-uterine devices[1] (Table 5.3).

MUR tips

Combined oral contraceptive

Menstrual bleeding is usually regular, lighter and less painful. Women with acne notice an improvement when using COCs. Breakthrough bleeding or spotting is common in the first few months of COC use. The COC can raise blood pressure in some women so this requires close monitoring.[1] A blood pressure check can be offered during the MUR.

- Reassure women who have concerns about fertility that this returns to normal after stopping the COC.[1]
- Check if women taking COCs are experiencing headaches or migraines.[1] Refer a patient to her GP if she presents with these symptoms.

- Check if women taking a COC are experiencing any unscheduled bleeding.[1] Refer to her GP if this is the case.
- Check that the patient is compliant with the COC and offer contraceptive measures advice if a pill(s) is missed. Reassure a woman who has missed one pill in the packet that she will not be putting herself at risk of pregnancy provided that:
  - she has taken all the other pills in the packet correctly
  - there has been nothing else that may have stopped her pill from working (e.g. vomiting, diarrhoea or interacting drug)
  - she has taken the final week of the last packet of pills correctly.[2]

Progestogen-only pill

This type of contraceptive is used when a COC is not suitable, e.g. heavy smokers, women with hypertension, women with migraine, older women (aged >35 years) and breastfeeding mothers. Menstrual irregularities are common with the POP but tend to resolve with time. Some women taking the POP may develop functional ovarian cysts.[1]

- A missed POP is one that is taken more than 3 hours late (or 12 hours in the case of Cerazette). Advise the patient to use additional contraceptive precautions for the next 2 days and to take the POP as soon as possible. Women should continue taking their pills daily.[1]

Combined contraceptive patch

The patch is replaced on a weekly basis. If a patient has vomiting or diarrhoea then contraceptive protection is not compromised, as the hormones are absorbed through the skin rather than the gastrointestinal tract. Some women may experience breast tenderness during the first couple of months of patch use,[1] so reassurance should be provided if this is the case.

- If a combined contraceptive patch detaches from its application site and has been off for less than 48 hours advise a patient to reapply it as soon as possible if it is still sticky. If a patch is not sticky then advise the patient to apply a new patch otherwise contraceptive protection will be compromised if a non-sticky patch is used.[1]

Long-acting progestogens

These are available as injectable preparations that provide contraception for a time period of a few months. This type of contraception is particularly suitable for young women and women with learning disabilities.[1]

- The most common adverse effects experienced by women taking long-acting progestogens is weight gain.[1] Invite the patient to have her weight monitored at the pharmacy.
- Some women may experience heavy or prolonged bleeding.[1] If this is the case, refer the patient to her GP, documenting this on the MUR form.

Intrauterine devices

There are two types: a copper intrauterine device (IUD) and a levonorgestrel-releasing IUD. IUDs provide contraceptive protection over a long period of time and are effective immediately after insertion. The levonorgestrel-releasing IUD can make periods lighter, shorter and less painful.[1]

Copper IUDs

These can cause heavy bleeding or bleeding between periods.[1] Patients experiencing pain can be recommended a suitable OTC analgesic or NSAID.

Levonorgestrel-releasing IUD

Abnormal bleeding is a problem with this IUD. One possible cause is misplacement of the device.[1] A patient should be referred to her GP if this is suspected.

Table 5.3 Examples of the types of contraception[3]

COCs	POPs	Combined contraceptive patch	Long-acting progestogens	IUDs
Loestrin 20 (low-strength COC)	Cerazette	Evra – currently a Black Triangle drug so report any adverse effects to the MHRA	Depo-Provera	Multiload Cu375 (copper IUD)
Microgynon 30	Femulen		Noristerat	MultiSafe 375 (copper IUD)
Ovranette	Micronor			Mirena (levonorgestrel IUD)
Cilest	Noriday			
BiNovum (biphasic COC)	Norgeston			
Logynon (triphasic COC)				

COC, combined oral contraceptives; IUD, intrauterine device; MHRA, Medical Health products Regulatory Authority; POP, progestogen-only pill.

Additional considerations

- Check that women who are taking an oral contraceptive are taking it correctly and consistently.[1]
- COC and POP effectiveness is reduced by drugs that induce liver enzymes (e.g. carbamazepine, phenytoin and topiramate). Antibacterials (e.g. ampicillin, doxycycline) alter bacterial flora that recycle ethinylestradiol from the bowel, so they will also reduce COC and POP effectiveness.[3] If a woman is taking an interacting drug, check that she is using additional contraceptive measures.
- Advise women who smoke to stop. Signpost smokers to a smoking cessation service.
- Advise women taking oestrogen containing contraceptives to stop taking them 4 weeks before major surgery.[3]

References

1. NHS Clinical Knowledge Summaries. Clinical Topic: Contraception. Available at: http://cks.library.nhs.uk/contraception (accessed 19 October 2009).
2. Family Planning Association (FPA). Contraception. Available at: www.fpa.org.uk (accessed 19 October 2009).
3. Joint Formulary Committee. *British National Formulary 57*. London: BMA and RPSGB, 2009.

6
Urinary tract conditions
Urinary incontinence

Condition

Incontinence is a condition of involuntary urinary leakage. It can be classified into stress incontinence, urge incontinence and overflow incontinence.[1]

Treatment options

Antimuscarinics and duloxetine.[1]

MUR tips

Antimuscarinics

Examples include oxybutynin, flavoxate, propiverine, tolterodine and trospium. Immediate-release oxybutynin is offered as first-line treatment.[2] Adverse effects associated with the use of antimuscarinics include dry mouth, blurred vision, drowsiness, dizziness and fatigue. Modified-release oxybutynin can be considered for those who find antimuscarinic adverse effects troublesome, but cost implications must be considered before this is routinely recommended.[2] Oxybutynin is also available as a transdermal patch or oral solution for patients experiencing difficulty in swallowing tablets. Antimuscarinics can be taken with or without food but trospium must be taken with a glass of water before meals or on an empty stomach.[1]

Duloxetine

This can be offered as an alternative to surgical treatment.[2] Duloxetine is commenced at a low dose to reduce discontinuation due to adverse effects.[1] Duloxetine commonly causes dry mouth, nausea and constipation in the first week of treatment.[3]

Additional considerations

- Pelvic floor muscle training exercises are recommended as first-line therapy for a period of 3 months.[2] Information for pharmacists on pelvic floor muscle exercises is available at www.netdoctor.co.uk/womenshealth/sui/pelvicfloor_005167.htm (accessed 19 October 2009). Patients can be given information on these exercises during the MUR.
- Patients should be advised to modify their fluid intake in order to alleviate symptoms of incontinence.[2]
- Patients with a BMI >30 should be advised to lose weight.[2] Patients can be invited to have their weight monitored at the pharmacy.
- Absorbent products, hand-held urinals and toilet aids can be used as an adjunct to ongoing treatment.[2]
- Patients with overflow incontinence should be advised to reduce their daily caffeine intake.[2]
- Advise patients to stop smoking. Signpost smokers to a smoking cessation service.

References

1. NHS Clinical Knowledge Summaries. Clinical Topic: Incontinence. Available at: http://cks.library.nhs.uk/draft_incontinence_urinary_in_women/background_information/definition#-368698. (accessed 1 February 2009).

2. National Institute for Health and Clinical Excellence. *Urinary Incontinence: The management of urinary incontinence in women: A quick reference guide.* NICE Guideline CG 40. London: NICE, 2006. Available at: www.nice.org.uk/nicemedia/pdf/word/CG40quickrefguide1006.pdf. (accessed 19 October 2009).
3. Electronic Medicines Compendium. Yentreve. Available at: http://emc.medicines.org.uk/ (accessed 19 October 2009).

Benign prostatic hyperplasia

Condition

A condition in which prostatic enlargement results in interference with normal urinary flow.

Treatment options

α Blockers and 5α-reductase inhibitors.[1]

MUR tips

α Blockers

These are usually the first drug of choice. Alfuzosin and tamsulosin are the best tolerated α blockers. Adverse effects tend to occur during the initial treatment period, most commonly dizziness, drowsiness, headache, postural hypotension and weakness. The risk of postural hypotension is reduced if the dose is taken at bedtime. Modified-release preparations are available for doxazosin, alfuzosin and tamsulosin, and may be considered for frail elderly men who may be more susceptible to first-dose postural hypotension.[1]

5α-Reductase inhibitors (finasteride)

These can be used in combination with α blockers. Adverse effects associated with use include decreased libido, ejaculation disorder and erectile dysfunction. The incidence of sexual adverse effects decreases with longer duration of treatment.[2]

Additional considerations

- The following factors may all aggravate the symptoms of benign prostatic hyperplasia (BPH): use of drugs with anticholinergic adverse effects (including over-the-counter [OTC] flu remedies or sedating antihistamines), constipation, alcohol and caffeine.[1] Advice on these can be given during the MUR.
- Advise men to relax when initiating voiding and to void twice to ensure that the bladder is emptied completely.[1]
- Advise men to retrain the bladder by increasing the intervals between emptying the bladder.[1] This will also increase the bladder's capacity.
- Information for pharmacists on Kegel Exercises for men is available at www.kegelexercisesformen.com/index.html (accessed 19 October 2009).

References

1. NHS Clinical Knowledge Summaries. Clinical Topic: Prostate benign hyperplasia. Available at: http://cks.library.nhs.uk/prostate_benign_ hyperplasia (accessed 19 October 2009).
2. Electronic Medicines Compendium. Proscar. Available at: http:// emc.medicines.org.uk/ (accessed 19 October 2009).

Chronic kidney disease

Condition

A progressive loss of nephrons resulting in deterioration of renal function.

Treatment options

These may include erythropoietins, phosphate-binding agents, hydroxylated vitamin D, oral sodium bicarbonate, antihypertensive agents, lipid-lowering agents and antiplatelet treatment.[1]

MUR tips

Erythropoietins

These are used to correct anaemia associated with erythropoietin deficiency. Proprietary examples include Eprex and Aranesp.[1] These products are available in pre-filled syringes, which require refrigeration. Check that patients are allowing the pre-filled syringe to reach room temperature before injecting. During the MUR explore how patients are injecting. Ensure that they are rotating the injection site and inject slowly to minimise discomfort at the injection site.[2]

Phosphate-binding agents

Examples include calcium acetate (Phosex) and sevelamer. Adverse effects associated with use include nausea and vomiting.[2] Check that the patient has regular blood tests to check serum phosphate and calcium levels. Patients should be advised to avoid purchasing calcium carbonate-based antacids (e.g. Rennie and Tums) in order to prevent hypercalcaemia.[2]

Hydroxylated vitamin D

Examples include alfacalcidol and calcitriol. Adverse effects associated with use result from hypercalcaemia and can manifest as nausea, vomiting and constipation.[1] If a patient reports any of these symptoms, refer to the GP, documenting this on the MUR form.

Oral sodium bicarbonate

This is used in cases of metabolic acidosis.[1,3] Check that the patient is having regular blood tests and advise him or her to avoid purchasing antacids that can disrupt acid–base balance.

Antihypertensive agents, lipid-lowering agents and antiplatelet treatments

See Chapter 2 for details.

Additional considerations

- Advise patients to monitor their intake of dietary protein.[4] Patients should be encouraged to have a low protein intake in their diet.[3]
- Patients should be given advice on dietary potassium, phosphate, calorie and salt intake.[4] Dietary intake of each should be low:

potassium (0.6 g/kg per day), phosphate (6.5 mg/kg per day) and low intake of water-soluble vitamins.[3]

- Advise patients to stop smoking.[3,4] Signpost smokers to a smoking cessation service.
- Encourage the patient to take regular aerobic exercise.[3]
- Alcohol consumption should be ≤3 units/day for men and ≤2 units/day for women.[3]
- Patients should be encouraged to maintain normal body weight (BMI <25).[3]
- Ensure that patients maintain strict blood pressure control. A blood pressure check can be offered during the MUR.
- Ensure that patients are aware of the potential for sodium retention with use of OTC NSAIDs and effervescent analgesic preparations that have a high sodium content.

References

1. Joint Formulary Committee. *British National Formulary 57*. London: BMA and RPSGB, 2009.
2. Electronic Medicines Compendium: Eprex, Aranesp, Phosex, Renagel. Available at: http://emc.medicines.org.uk/ (accessed 19 October 2009).
3. GP Notebook. Chronic renal disease. Available at: www.gpnotebook.co.uk (accessed 19 October 2009).
4. National Institute for Health and Clinical Excellence. *Chronic Kidney Disease: A quick reference guide*. NICE Guideline CG 73. London: NICE, 2008. Available at: www.nice.org.uk/nicemedia/pdf/CG073QuickRefGuide.pdf. (accessed 19 October 2009).

7
Haematological conditions

Iron deficiency anaemia

Condition

A condition where low levels of iron in the blood can lead to anaemia. This may give rise to symptoms such as breathlessness, pallor and tiredness.

Treatment options

Iron supplements.[1,2]

MUR tips

Iron supplements include ferrous sulphate, ferrous fumarate and ferrous gluconate. Iron replacement usually requires between 120 mg and 180 mg of elemental iron per day, and the amount of elemental iron varies according to the preparation[2] (Table 7.1). Common adverse effects associated with use are nausea, constipation, diarrhoea, black faeces and abdominal discomfort.[3]

Table 7.1 Elemental iron content for iron preparations available[3]

Preparation	Iron salt	Amount of iron salt (mg) per dose unit	Amount of elemental iron (mg)
Ferrous Sulphate	Ferrous sulphate	200	65
Ferrograd	Ferrous sulphate	325	105
Fersaday	Ferrous fumarate	322	100
Fersamal	Ferrous fumarate	210	68
Galfer	Ferrous fumarate	305	100
Ferrous Gluconate	Ferrous gluconate	300	35
Sytron elixir	Sodium feredetate	190	27.5 mg/5mL

Additional considerations

- During the MUR assess compliance because non-compliance may lead to inadequate treatment.
- During the MUR advise patients to have a balanced intake of iron-rich foods such as spinach, meat, lentils, apricots, prunes and raisins.[1,2]

- Check that patients regularly attend appointments for blood tests and monitor the length of the iron treatment course. Once the patient's haemoglobin concentration is normal, iron supplementation should be continued for 3 months and can then be stopped, with appropriate monitoring.[1]
- During the MUR ensure that patients are aware of the food types that can increase and decrease iron absorption (Table 7.2).
- During the MUR remind patients to take the iron supplement with or after meals. This helps to minimise the adverse effects that may be experienced.[1]
- Patients experiencing black stools during the treatment course can be reassured that the cause is likely to be the iron supplement.
- Patients who experience intolerable adverse effects from the iron preparation prescribed may benefit from taking a different iron salt (e.g. ferrous gluconate) with a lower amount of elemental iron.[1] This recommendation can be made on the MUR form for the GP to consider.
- Modified preparations are formulated to release iron in the small bowel where iron is not absorbed. Therefore, there is no therapeutic advantage to modified-release preparations.[1,3]
- Over-the-counter (OTC) antacids can reduce the absorption of iron supplements.[3] Check that patients are aware of this and advise them to avoid taking antacids at the same time as iron supplements.

Table 7.2 Examples of foods that increase or decrease iron absorption[1,2]

Foods increasing iron absorption	Foods decreasing iron absorption
Vitamin C	Phytates, e.g. wholegrain cereals, chapatti flour, nuts and seeds
Fish (high intake required)	Tea and coffee

Table 7.2 *Continued*

Foods increasing iron absorption	Foods decreasing iron absorption
Red meat (high intake required)	Calcium from dairy products
White meat (high intake required)	Antacids containing zinc and magnesium salts

References

1. NHS Clinical Knowledge Summaries. Clinical Topic: Iron Deficiency Anaemia. Available at: http://cks.library.nhs.uk/anaemia_iron_deficiency (accessed 19 October 2009).
2. GP Notebook. Iron deficiency anaemia. Available at: http://www.gpnotebook.co.uk/simplepage.cfm?ID=1993342985 (accessed 19 October 2009).
3. Joint Formulary Committee. *British National Formulary 57.* London: BMA and RPSGB, 2009.

Pernicious anaemia

Condition

An autoimmune condition in which there is deficiency of intrinsic factor. This results in vitamin B_{12} deficiency, causing megaloblastic anaemia.

Treatment options

Hydroxocobalamin and folic acid.[1]

> ### MUR tips
>
> #### Hydroxocobalamin
>
> The initial treatment course is 1 mg intramuscularly three times a week for 2 weeks then 1 mg every 3 months.[1,2] During the MUR, check the frequency with which the patient is attending appointments for injections. Adverse effects associated with use may include nausea, vomiting, diarrhoea and headache.[3]
>
> #### Folic acid
>
> An oral dose of 5 mg daily is used. Most patients require treatment for 4 months, although some may need to take it on a long-term basis.[1]

Additional considerations

- Advise patients to eat foods rich in vitamin B_{12}, e.g. breakfast cereals and breads fortified with vitamin B_{12}.[1]
- Advise patients to eat foods rich in folic acid, e.g. broccoli, Brussels sprouts, peas, chickpeas and brown rice.[1]
- During the MUR check how often patients are attending for blood tests and monitor the length of the treatment course.

References

1. NHS Clinical Knowledge Summaries. Clinical Topic: Pernicious anaemia. Available at: http://cks.library.nhs.uk/anaemia_b12_and_folate_deficiency (accessed 19 October 2009).
2. Joint Formulary Committee. *British National Formulary 57*. London: BMA and RPSGB, 2009.
3. Electronic Medicines Compendium. Neo-cytamen injection. Available at: http://emc.medicines.org.uk/ (accessed 19 October 2009).

8
Bone and joint disorders
Rheumatoid arthritis

Condition

A progressive inflammatory condition of the small joints which can result in pain, deformity and impairment of function.

Treatment options

Paracetamol, codeine, NSAIDs, corticosteroids and disease-modifying antirheumatic drugs (DMARDs).[1]

MUR tips

Paracetamol

This is an effective painkiller for mild-to-moderate pain. It is more effective when used regularly than on an 'as-required' basis.[1] Patients may commonly feel that paracetamol is ineffective but often they may not be taking a therapeutic dose. Explore patients' use of paracetamol during the MUR.

Codeine

This is added separately rather than in combination with paracetamol. Codeine can provide additional pain relief if used with paracetamol. Adverse effects associated with use may include nausea, vomiting, constipation and drowsiness. Constipation can be a problem for some patients, who may require regular laxative use.[1]

NSAIDs

Examples include ibuprofen, diclofenac and naproxen. Adverse effects associated with use include gastrointestinal adverse effects, worsening of asthma and renal impairment.[1,2] Refer patients experiencing dyspepsia to the GP for consideration of the addition of a gastroprotective agent, documenting this on the MUR form.

Corticosteroids

Oral corticosteroids are not recommended for regular use.[3] Short courses at the lowest possible dose for the shortest period of time are used during flare-ups.[2,3] Adverse effects associated with use include hypertension, cataracts, osteoporosis and thinning of the skin.[1]

DMARDs

Several DMARDs are used, each requiring specific considerations during the MUR (Table 8.1). Sulfasalazine and methotrexate are the DMARDs of choice due to their favourable efficacy and toxicity profiles.[3]

Table 8.1 Examples of disease-modifying antirheumatic drugs (DMARDs) and points for discussion during the MUR[1]

DMARD	Specific considerations for discussion during the MUR
Azathioprine	Requires regular monitoring throughout the treatment course.[1] Signs of azathioprine toxicity include rashes, oral ulceration, abnormal bruising or severe sore throats.[1] Patients who report any of these symptoms should be advised to see their GP as soon as possible.
Ciclosporin	Signs of ciclosporin toxicity include abnormal bruising.[1] During the MUR check whether the patient experiences this and encourage immediate advice from the GP should this be the case. Blood pressure can be elevated during treatment.[1] A blood pressure-monitoring service can be offered to patients. If their blood pressure is persistently high the patient should be referred to the GP for review of treatment.
Hydroxychloroquine	Adverse effects associated with use may include blurred vision and changes in visual acuity. Annual appointments with the optometrist are advised[1] and the MUR is an opportunity to check whether the patient attends for these appointments.
Leflunomide	Adverse effects associated with use include rashes, hair loss, abnormal bruising, severe sore throat, weight loss, hypertension and breathlessness.[1] Patients can be offered a blood pressure-monitoring service at the pharmacy. Patients should also be encouraged to report any adverse effects immediately and referred to their GP for review of their treatment.

Table 8.1 *Continued*

DMARD	Specific considerations for discussion during the MUR
Penicillamine	Adverse effects associated with use include severe rash, oral ulceration, nausea, taste alteration, abnormal bruising and severe sore throat.[1] Patients should be encouraged to report any adverse effects immediately and be referred to the GP for review of their treatment.
Sulfasalazine	Adverse effects associated with use may include widespread rash, oral ulceration, nausea, headache, abnormal bruising and severe sore throat.[1] Patients should be encouraged to report any adverse effects immediately and be referred to the GP for review of their treatment.
Methotrexate	During the MUR check that the patient is taking methotrexate on a weekly basis. Patients may also be taking folic acid tablets, so it is advisable to check that they are able to differentiate between the two.[4] Adverse effects associated with use include rash, oral ulceration, nausea, vomiting, severe sore throat, abnormal bruising, dry persistent cough and breathlessness.[1,4] Patients should be encouraged to report any adverse effects immediately and be referred to the GP for review of their treatment.

Additional considerations

* Encourage patients to take regular non-weight-bearing exercise such as swimming to improve joint flexibility.[2]
* Encourage patients to eat a Mediterranean-style diet.[2]
* Patients may benefit from assistive devices such as walking sticks and tap turners. Signpost patients to device providers during the MUR.

References

1. NHS Clinical Knowledge Summaries. Clinical Topic: Rheumatoid Arthritis. Available at: http://cks.library.nhs.uk/rheumatoid_arthritis (accessed 19 October 2009).
2. National institute for Health and Clinical Excellence. *Rheumatoid Arthritis: The management of rheumatoid arthritis in adults: A quick reference guide.* NICE Guideline CG 79. London: NICE, 2009. Available at: www.nice.org.uk/nicemedia/pdf/CG79QuickRefGuide.pdf. (accessed 19 October 2009).
3. Scottish Intercollegiate Guidelines Network. *Management of Early Rheumatoid Arthritis, Quick reference guide.* SIGN Guideline 48. Edinburgh: SIGN, 2000. Available at: www.sign.ac.uk/pdf/qrg48.pdf. (accessed 19 October 2009).
4. National Patient Safety Agency (NPSA). *Guidelines on Improving Compliance with Oral Methotrexate.* London: NPSA, 2006. Available at: www.npsa.nhs.uk/nrls/alerts-and-directives/alerts/oral-methotrexate/. (accessed 19 October 2009).

Osteoarthritis

Condition

A degenerative condition of the joints giving rise to joint pain. Commonly known as 'wear and tear' of the joints.

Treatment options

Paracetamol and topical NSAIDs.[1,2]

MUR tips

Paracetamol

This is an effective painkiller for mild-to-moderate pain. It is more effective when used regularly rather than on an 'as-required' basis.[1] Patients may commonly feel that paracetamol is ineffective but often may not be taking a therapeutic dose. Explore patients' use of paracetamol during the MUR.

Topical NSAIDs

These include ibuprofen gel which is suitable for people with knee or hand osteoarthritis. A combination of paracetamol and topical NSAIDs is offered before oral NSAIDs are considered.[2] During the MUR check that patients are using topical products appropriately to gain maximum benefit.

Additional considerations

- Patients should be advised to do muscle-strengthening exercises, such as walking, to improve their aerobic fitness.[1,2]
- Patients should be advised to lose weight if they are overweight or obese.[1,2] Invite patients to have their weight monitored at the pharmacy.
- Some patients may benefit from a transcutaneous electrical nerve stimulation (TENS) machine.[2] More information on the use of a TENS machine can be provided in the MUR.
- Patients with hip osteoarthritis may benefit from manipulation and stretching exercises.[2]
- Patients may benefit from assistive devices such as walking sticks and tap turners.[2] Signpost patients to device providers during the MUR.

References

1. NHS Clinical Knowledge Summaries. Clinical Topic: Osteoarthritis. http://cks.library.nhs.uk/osteoarthritis (accessed 19 October 2009).
2. National Institute for Health and Clinical Excellence. *Osteoarthritis: A quick reference guide.* NICE Guideline CG 59. London: NICE, 2008. Available at: www.nice.org.uk/nicemedia/pdf/CG59quickrefguide.pdf (accessed 19 October 2009).

Osteoporosis

Condition

A condition of low bone mineral density resulting in an increased risk of bone fractures.

Treatment options

Bisphosphonate, strontium ranelate and calcium + vitamin D.[1]

MUR tips

Bisphosphonate

Examples include alendronate, etidronate and risedronate. Alendronate is the first treatment of choice[2] and can be taken as a daily or once-weekly dose. Check that patients are taking once-weekly alendronate 30 min before breakfast with a full glass of plain water (mineral water may reduce the absorption of alendronate). They should not lie down for at least 30 min after taking alendronate in order to reduce gastrointestinal adverse effects such as dyspepsia, acid regurgitation and constipation.[1,3] Other bisphosphonates are also administered in this way.

Strontium ranelate

This is an alternative to bisphosphonates if patients cannot comply with the administration instructions for bisphosphonates.[1,2] The preparation is available as a powder sachet which is taken as a suspension in a glass of water. It must be taken at bedtime at least 2 hours after the evening meal.[3] During the MUR check the patient's use of this product and explore any adverse effects that he or she may be experiencing.

Calcium + vitamin D

Patients should aim to have a good dietary intake of calcium + vitamin D (Table 8.2). Patients should aim to take 700 mg calcium and 400 IU vitamin D daily. Supplementation may be required to achieve these recommended levels.[1]

Table 8.2 Dietary sources rich in calcium and vitamin D[1,4]

Calcium	1000 mg calcium can be obtained from: 1 pint (600 mL) milk 60 g Edam or cheddar cheese, 125 g yoghurt. Other foods that are a good source of calcium include spinach, watercress, dried apricots, dried figs and white bread.
Vitamin D	400 IU vitamin D can be obtained from 120 g cooked salmon or cooked mackerel.

Additional considerations

- Bisphosphonates: during the MUR check that patients are adhering to the administration instructions for bisphosphonates.

Patients experiencing gastrointestinal adverse effects should be given advice on alleviating these by correct use of the product.

- The absorption of bisphosphonates can be impaired by calcium supplements and antacids. Patients should be advised to wait at least 30 min after taking a bisphosphonate before taking any other oral medication.[3]
- Patients who smoke should be advised to stop smoking. Smoking can increase the risk of osteoporosis.[4] Signpost patients to a smoking cessation service.
- Patients should be encouraged to undertake low-impact weight-bearing exercises such as walking.[1]

References

1. NHS Clinical Knowledge Summaries. Clinical Topic: Osteoporosis. Available at: http://cks.library.nhs.uk/osteoporosis_treatment (accessed 19 October 2009).
2. National Institute for Health and Clinical Excellence. *Osteoporosis: Secondary prevention including strontium ranelate: A quick reference guide*. NICE Guideline TA 161. London: NICE, 2008. Available at: www.nice.org.uk/nicemedia/pdf/TA161quickrefguide.pdf (accessed 19 October 2009).
3. Electronic Medicines Compendium Fosamax and Protelos. Available at: http://emc.medicines.org.uk (accessed 19 October 2009).
4. Scottish Intercollegiate Guidelines Network. *Management of Osteoporosis, guideline*. SIGN Guideline 71. Edinburgh: SIGN, 2003. Available at: www.sign.ac.uk/pdf/sign71.pdf (accessed 19 October 2009).

Gout

Condition

A condition resulting in joint pain and inflammation due to high serum uric acid levels. The big toe is commonly affected first.

Treatment options

NSAIDs, colchicine and allopurinol.[1,2]

MUR tips

NSAIDs

Examples include naproxen and diclofenac. Adverse effects associated with use include gastrointestinal adverse effects, worsening of asthma and renal impairment.[1] Refer patients experiencing dyspepsia to their GP for consideration of a gastroprotective agent, documenting this on the MUR form.

Colchicine

This is taken during an acute attack of gout at a dose of 6 mg per course (often 500 mcg taken four times a day for 3 days). The course of treatment during an acute attack should not be repeated within 3 days of the previous course.[1,2] Common adverse effects include nausea, vomiting and abdominal pain.[3]

Allopurinol

Maintenance doses are usually 300 mg/day but some patients may require doses in the range of 100–900 mg daily depending on the severity of their condition.[1] A common adverse effect associated with use is skin reactions.[1,3] If patients complain of a rash during treatment with allopurinol, refer them to the GP, documenting this on the MUR form.

Additional considerations

- Patients should be advised to restrict the amount of foods rich in purines in their diet. Foods containing large amounts of purines include red meat, liver, yeast extracts, shellfish, cauliflower, spinach and mushrooms.[1]
- Advise patients to avoid consumption of alcoholic beverages such as stout, beer, port and fortified wines, because they can precipitate an attack of gout.[1]
- Advise patients to consume 2 litres of water a day.[1] This helps to prevent the build-up of uric acid crystals in the joints.
- Patients should be encouraged to maintain a normal body weight (BMI <25).[1] Patients can be invited to have their weight monitored at the pharmacy.
- Advise patients to take regular exercise (e.g. swimming) and to avoid intense exercise types that may cause trauma to joints.[1]

References:

1. NHS Clinical Knowledge Summaries. Clinical Topic: Gout. Available at: http://cks.library.nhs.uk/gout (accessed 19 October 2009).
2. Joint Formulary Committee. *British National Formulary 57*. London: BMA and RPSGB, 2009.
3. Electronic Medicines Compendium. Colchicine and Zyloric. Available at: http://emc.medicines.org.uk/ (accessed 19 October 2009).

9
Eye conditions

Glaucoma

Condition

An eye condition characterised by raised intraocular pressure, resulting in loss of sight.

Treatment options

β Blockers, prostaglandin analogues and carbonic anhydrase inhibitors.[1]

MUR tips

β Blockers

Those used include levobunolol and timolol. Adverse effects associated with use include hypotension, bronchospasm, nausea and headaches.[2] Explore any difficulties that the patient may experience with administering the eye drops.

Prostaglandin analogues

These are often the drug of first choice.[3] Examples include latanoprost, travoprost and bimatoprost. Adverse effects associated with use include iris pigmentation and eyelash growth.[2] During the MUR check that patients who use latanoprost are adhering to the refrigeration storage requirements of the product.

Carbonic anhydrase inhibitors

These include brinzolamide and dorzolamide. Adverse effects associated with use include dry mouth and headache.[2]

Additional considerations

- Check that patients discard any eye drop bottles 28 days after opening.[3] During the MUR explore how patients keep track of the length of time for which eye drop bottles have been open.
- Eye drops can cause local adverse effects such as stinging, blurred vision, pain, itching and dry eyes.[1,3]
- During the MUR check that the patient is administering only one drop to the eye at any one time, because administering several drops at a time may increase the risk of adverse effects.[3]
- Check that patients close the eye after application of the eye drop without tightly squeezing the eyelids.[3]
- Check that patients who are using more than one type of eye drop are allowing a 5-minute interval between applying the first eye drop and the second.[3]
- If a patient has one short-acting and one long-acting eye drop, check that he or she is putting the long-acting eye drop in last.[3]
- If a patient wears soft contact lenses, check that they are removing the lenses before applying the eye drops and are waiting at least 15 min before putting the lenses back in.[3]
- Check that the patient attends for regular eye tests.
- Elderly patients or those with poor eyesight may benefit from a combination product.[3] This suggestion can be documented on the action points section of the MUR form, for the prescriber to consider.

- Patients who have difficulties in administering their eye drops may benefit from using an Opticare device (Figure 9.1). The use of this device can be demonstrated during the MUR.

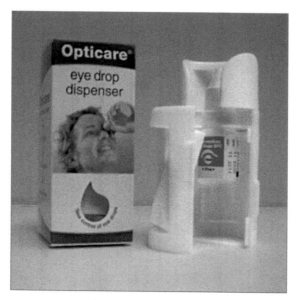

Figure 9.1   Opticare device.

References

1. Joint Formulary Committee. *British National Formulary 57*. London: BMA and RPSGB, 2009.
2. Electronic Medicines Compendium: Betagan, Lumigan, Xalatan, Azopt. Available at: http://emc.medicines.org.uk (accessed 19 October 2009).
3. National Prescribing Centre. Recent developments in primary open angle glaucoma and ocular hypertension. *MeReC Bull* 2003; 13 (5):17–20. Available at: www.npc.co.uk/ebt/merec/therap/other/resources/merec_bulletin_vol13_no5.pdf (accessed 19 October 2009).

Dry eyes

Condition

A disorder of the tear film leaving eyes dry, with a feeling of discomfort.

Treatment options

Artificial tears and ocular lubricants.[1]

MUR tips

Artificial tears and ointments

Hypromellose is the most commonly used product but requires frequent administration. Carbomers (e.g. Viscotears, GelTears) and polyvinyl alcohol (e.g. Sno Tears) are longer acting.[1]

Ocular lubricants

Paraffin-based ointments (e.g. Lacri-Lube) are applied at night and can cause blurring of vision.[1]

Additional considerations

- Dry eyes result from an adverse effect of other prescribed medication that patients may be taking, e.g. antihistamines, selective serotonin reuptake inhibitors (SSRIs).[1]
- During the MUR, check if patients are experiencing eye irritation. The preservative benzalkonium chloride, which is found in eye drops, can be the cause of this.[1] In this case a preservative-free product can be recommended and the suggestion for a change to the patient's prescription can be documented on the MUR form.
- Check that patients are discarding their eye drop bottles 1 month after opening.
- Contact lenses should be avoided if the patient experiences dry eyes.
- Patients who use the computer for long periods of time may develop dry eyes. Advise patients to take regular breaks and to avoid staring at the computer screen.[1]
- Smoking can cause dry eyes.[1] Signpost smokers to a smoking cessation service.

Reference

1. NHS Clinical Knowledge Summaries. Clinical Topic: Dry Eyes. Available at: http://cks.library.nhs.uk/dry_eye_syndrome (accessed 19 October 2009).

10
Skin conditions

Eczema

Condition

A skin condition resulting in dry, red and itchy skin.

Treatment options

Emollients and topical corticosteroids.[1]

MUR tips

Emollients

Ointments are prescribed for extremely dry skin whereas creams and lotions are used on skin that is less dry. Encourage patients to apply emollients frequently throughout the day.[1] Ointments are often cosmetically unacceptable compared with creams which are the preferred choice for regular application during the day.[4] A common adverse effect associated with use is skin sensitivity to an ingredient in the emollient.[1] In this instance advise patients to try another emollient after a comprehensive discussion in the MUR.

Topical corticosteroids

The potency of the topical corticosteroid prescribed depends on the severity of the eczema (Table 10.1). The likelihood of adverse effects occurring depends on the potency and the amount of topical corticosteroid used. Adverse effects include a transient burning or stinging of the skin.[1] Topical corticosteroids are used to control flare-ups and their use should be limited to a treatment period of 3–7 days.[2] Topical corticosteroids should be applied thinly on the skin. Remind patients that one fingertip unit (approximately 500 mg) is enough to cover the area of two flat adult palms.[3] During the MUR explore how the patient is using their topical corticosteroid and if they adhere to the fingertip unit rule.

Table 10.1 The potency of available corticosteroid preparations[3]

Topical corticosteroid	Potency
Hydrocortisone 0.1–2.5%	Mild
Betamethasone valerate 0.025%, Clobetasone butyrate 0.05%	Moderate
Betamethasone valerate 0.1%, Fluocinolone acetonide 0.025%, Hydrocortisone butyrate 0.1%, Mometasone furoate 0.1%	Potent
Clobetasol propionate 0.05%	Very potent

Reproduced from the BNF. The reader is reminded that the BNF is constantly revised so for the latest guidelines please consult the current edition of the BNF.

Additional considerations

- Contact emollient manufacturers to obtain sample packs to provide patients with a range to try. This allows patients to find a suitable emollient that they will feel able to use frequently. A variety of emollients is available (Table 10.2 and Figure 10.1) (see website www.eczema.org).
- Check that patients are applying emollients frequently throughout the day.[1] Table 10.3 shows the weekly amount of emollients that can be applied on adults based on a twice-daily application.[3]
- Check that patients are being prescribed sufficient quantities of emollients. The patient should be using at least 10 times more emollient than topical corticosteroid.[1] If a patient has insufficient quantities prescribed, suggest that quantities are increased on repeat prescriptions and document this on the action plan section of the MUR form.
- Encourage patients to carry a small-sized pack of emollient with them for regular use during the day.
- Check that patients are applying emollients gently in the direction of hair growth rather than rubbing them in vigorously (see www.eczema.org). This minimises skin aggravation.
- Check that patients continue to use their emollient after flare-ups have settled down. This helps to prevent further flare-ups (see www.eczema.org).
- Emollient bath additives and shower gels can be considered for those with extensive areas of dry skin. They should be used in addition to emollient ointments or creams.[1]
- Advise patients to monitor the number of flare-ups that they have and monitor the quantity of topical corticosteroid prescribed and used.
- Patients who use both a topical corticosteroid and an emollient should be advised to leave at least 15 min between applications of each product (see www.eczema.org). The topical corticosteroid should be applied first.
- Advise patients to avoid exacerbating factors such as wearing clothes containing wool or synthetic fibres and the use of certain soaps or detergents.[2]

- Advise patients to keep their nails short to avoid scratching.[2]
- Education is a key principle for the successful management of eczema. Provide patients with leaflets on their condition and demonstrations of correct emollient and topical corticosteroid use.[2]

Table 10.2 Examples of the emollients available

Lotions	Creams	Oint-ments	Gels	Soap substitutes	Bath oils	Shower products
Aveeno	Aveeno	50:50 white soft paraffin/ liquid paraffin	Double-base	Aqueous cream	Balneum and Balneum plus	Dermal 200
Dermal 500	Balneum plus	Emul-sifying ointment	Oilatum gel	Cetraben wash	Dermal 600	E45 shower
Eucerin lotion	Cetraben	Epaderm		E45 wash	Diprobath	Oilatum shower
Oilatum	Diprobase	Hydromol		Emulsi-fying ointment	Oilatum fragrance free	
E45 lotion	E45 cream	Hydrous ointment				

Table 10.3 Suitable weekly amount of emollients to be applied on an adult based on a twice-daily application[3]

Area of the body	Amount of cream and ointment to be applied (g)	Amount of lotion to be applied (mL)
Face	15–30	100
Both hands	25–50	200
Scalp	50–100	200
Both arms or both legs	100–200	200
Trunk	400	500
Groins and genitalia	15–25	100

Reproduced from the BNF. The reader is reminded that the BNF is constantly revised, so for the latest guidelines please consult the current edition of the BNF.

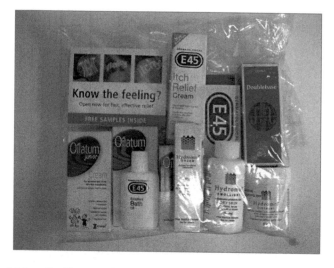

Figure 10.1   Emollient samples.

References

1. NHS Clinical Knowledge Summaries. Clinical Topic: Atopic Eczema. Available at: http://cks.library.nhs.uk/eczema_atopic (accessed 19 October 2009).
2. National Prescribing Centre. Atopic eczema in primary care. *MeReC Bull* 2003; 14(1):1–4. Available at: www.npc.co.uk/ebt/merec/therap/skin/resources/merec_bulletin_vol14_no1.pdf (accessed 19 October 2009).
3. Joint Formulary Committee. *British National Formulary 57*. London: BMA and RPSGB, 2009.

Psoriasis

Condition

A skin condition characterised by white/silvery skin plaques.

Treatment options

Vitamin D analogues, coal tar, dithranol and tazarotene.[1]

MUR tips

Vitamin D analogues

Examples include calcipotriol and tacalcitol. Vitamin D analogues are first-line treatments because they are odour free and do not stain.[1] Adverse effects associated with use may include skin irritation, burning and a stinging sensation on application.[2] Calcipotriol requires a fairly thick application layer compared with topical corticosteroids.[3] Check that patients are adhering to the correct method of administration.

Coal tar preparations

Proprietary examples include Clinitar, Exorex and Polytar. Proprietary coal tar preparations are less effective, taking longer for improvement in the psoriasis.[1] Adverse effects associated with use may include skin irritation and skin photosensitivity.[2]

Dithranol

Proprietary examples include Dithrocream and Micanol. Common adverse effects associated with use may include skin irritation on application and staining of the skin or hair.[2] Patients should be advised to wash off the proprietary 1–2% preparation 5–60 min after application.[1] During the MUR explore the patients' use of the product and ensure that correct administration is adhered to.

Tazarotene

Commonly experienced adverse effects include burning and skin irritation.[2] The Psoriasis Association recommend that patients apply Vaseline onto the plaques and surrounding skin 1 hour before applying tazarotene. This is thought to reduce the chance of skin irritation occurring (see www.psoriasis-association.org.uk).

Additional considerations

- Check that the patient is adhering to the correct method of administration for the product prescribed. If the patient is unsure, provide education and signpost the patient to support groups.
- Encourage patient to use emollients regularly.[3] See earlier for details on emollient use.

References

1. Joint Formulary Committee. *British National Formulary 57*. London: BMA and RPSGB, 2009.

2. Electronic Medicines Compendium. Dovonex, Exorex, Dithrocream, Zorac. Available at: http://emc.medicines.org.uk (accessed 19 October 2009).

3. Clark CM. Psoriasis: first-time treatments. *Pharm J* 2005; 274: 623–6.

Acne

Condition

A skin condition in which the hair follicle and sebaceous glands are implicated. Excessive production of sebum can result in pores becoming blocked. This results in the appearance of blackheads and whiteheads.

Treatment options

Benzoyl peroxide, topical antibiotics, topical retinoids, azelaic acid and oral antibiotics.[1,2]

MUR tips

Benzoyl peroxide

This is effective for mild-to-moderate acne.[2] Common adverse effects associated with use may include a mild burning sensation on first application and reddening and peeling of the skin.[3] Adverse effects usually subside with continued use of the product and less frequent applications.[2] Patients should be warned that benzoyl peroxide preparations can cause bleaching of hair, dyed fabrics and clothing.[1,3] During the MUR check that the patient is applying a thin layer of the product in order to minimise skin irritation.

Topical antibiotics

Examples include clindamycin and erythromycin. Topical antibiotics are less irritant than benzoyl peroxide.[4] Check that patients who use Zineryt are discarding the bottle 5 weeks after the dispensing date.[3] The main limitation of topical antibiotics is bacterial resistance rather than actual adverse effects.[1] During the MUR explore patients' perceptions of treatment efficacy.

Topical retinoids

These include tretinoin, isotretinoin and adapalene. Patients should be encouraged to continue using the product because it may take several months of treatment before a response is achieved.[2] One adverse effect is skin irritation, which improves with continued use of the product. Topical retinoids can cause skin sensitivity to ultraviolet light. Patients should be advised to limit their exposure to sunlight and sunlamps or to use a sunscreen product.[1,4]

Azelaic acid

This causes less skin irritation than benzoyl peroxide and topical retinoids.[1] Skin irritation often occurs at the start of treatment and subsides during the course of treatment.[3]

Oral antibiotics

Examples include oxytetracycline, tetracycline, minocycline and doxycycline. A rapid improvement in acne is observed within 2 weeks.[1] Maximal improvement in the condition is often achieved after 4–6 months of treatment. Some patients may require oral antibiotics for 2 years or more.[4]

Additional considerations

- Check that patients are applying a small amount of the topical products. Patients may expect quick results with treatments and may feel disappointed if that is not achieved. Patients are more likely to experience adverse effects earlier in the treatment course if large amounts of the topical product are applied. Education about the correct method of administration of the products can be provided during the MUR.
- Patients using topical preparations should be advised to apply the product to the 'spots' and adjacent areas to prevent development of new 'spots'.[4]
- Patients should be advised to avoid the use of abrasive cleansers and vigorous scrubbing as this may worsen the skin inflammation.[4]
- Advise patients to avoid 'picking the spots' because this may leave scars on the skin.[1]
- Dispel any misconceptions that patients may have about a link between acne and diet. There is no evidence that chocolate or fatty foods cause acne.[1]
- Advise patients to avoid wearing make-up if possible, but if it must be worn suggest that a light product be used.[1]
- Advise patients to avoid using ointments or oil-rich creams because they may clog the skin pores, with the potential of exacerbating acne.[1]
- Patients taking oral contraceptives who start taking oral antibiotics should be advised to use additional contraceptive precautions for the first 3 weeks.[2]

References

1. NHS Clinical Knowledge Summaries. Clinical Topic: Acne Vulgaris. Available at: http://cks.library.nhs.uk/acne_vulgaris (accessed 19 October 2009).
2. Joint Formulary Committee. *British National Formulary 57*. London: BMA and RPSGB, 2009.

3. Electronic Medicines Compendium. Panoxyl, Zineryt, Skinoren. Available at: http://emc.medicines.org.uk (accessed 19 October 2009).

4. National Prescribing Centre. The treatment of acne vulgaris: an update *MeReC Bull* 1999; 10(8):1–4. Available at: www.npc.co.uk/ebt/merec/therap/skin/resources/merec_bulletin_vol10_no08 pdf.(accessed 19 October 2009).

Index